Lange Instant Access
Acid-Base, Fluids, and Electrolytes

KU-370-206

Robert F. Reilly, Jr., MD

Fredric L. Coe Professor of Nephrolithiasis Research in Mineral Metabolism
Chief, Section of Nephrology
Veterans Affairs North Texas Health Care System
Professor of Medicine
Department of Medicine
The Charles and Jane Pak Center for Mineral Metabolism and Clinical Research
The University of Texas Southwestern Medical Center at Dallas
Dallas, Texas

Mark A. Perazella, MD, FACP

Associate Professor of Medicine
Director, Renal Fellowship Program
Director, Acute Dialysis Services
Section of Nephrology
Department of Medicine
Yale University School of Medicine
New Haven, Connecticut

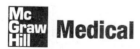 Medical

New York Chicago San Francisco Lisbon London
Madrid Mexico City Milan New Delhi San Juan Seoul
Singapore Sydney Toronto

The McGraw·Hill Companies

Lange Instant Access: Acid-Base, Fluids, and Electrolytes

1 2 3 4 5 6 7 8 9 0 DOC/DOC 0 9 8 7

ISBN-13: 978-0-07-148634-7
ISBN-10: 0-07-148634-8

This book was set in Times New Roman by International Typesetting and Composition, Inc.
The editors were Jim Shanahan, Maya Barahona, and Peter J. Boyle.
The production supervisor was Sherri Souffrance.
Project management was provided by International Typesetting and Composition, Inc.
RR Donnelley was the printer and binder.
This book is printed on acid-free paper.

Library of Congress Cataloging-in-Publication Data
Reilly, Robert F., M.D.
  Acid-base, fluids and electrolytes/Robert F. Reilly Jr., Mark A. Perazella.—1st ed.
      p. ; cm.—(Lange instant access)
  Includes bibliographical references and index.
  ISBN-13: 978-0-07-148634-7 (softcover : alk. paper)
  ISBN-10: 0-07-148634-8 (softcover : alk. paper) 1. Water-electrolyte imbalances. 2. Acid-based imbalances. I. Perazella, Mark A. II. Title. III. Series.
  [DNLM: 1. Acid-Base Imbalance—metabolism. 2. Body Fluids. 3. Water-Electrolyte Imbalance—metabolism. WD 220 R362a 2008]
RC630.A2357 2008
616.3'992—dc22
                              2007008918

To my wife Sheli, my parents Robert Sr. and Nancy, my son Rob, and my brothers Steven and Fred, whose help and support are invaluable in both my life and career. Also to Marc Siegelaub and Brad Thomas, who taught me the value of creative thinking, and to Stephen Colbert who covers all the bases without acidity.

Robert F. Reilly, Jr.

To my parents Joseph and Santina, whose guidance made my career in medicine possible, my brothers Joe and Scott, who are a constant source of encouragement, my wife Donna, whose unselfish support allowed me to undertake this project, and my sons Mark and Andrew, who bring boundless joy into my life. Also to my good friends Mark Albini and John Magaldi, who made the trek through medicine an interesting and unforgettable experience.

Mark A. Perazella

Contents

Contributors

Dinkar Kaw, MD
Assistant Professor of Medicine
Division of Nephrology
Department of Medicine
The University of Toledo College of Medicine
Toledo, Ohio

Mark A. Perazella, MD, FACP
Associate Professor of Medicine
Director, Renal Fellowship Program
Director, Acute Dialysis Services
Section of Nephrology
Department of Medicine
Yale University School of Medicine
New Haven, Connecticut

Robert F. Reilly, Jr., MD
Fredric L. Coe Professor of Nephrolithiasis Research
  in Mineral Metabolism
Chief, Section of Nephrology
Veterans Affairs North Texas Health Care System
Professor of Medicine
Department of Medicine
The Charles and Jane Pak Center for Mineral Metabolism
  and Clinical Research
The University of Texas Southwestern Medical Center
  at Dallas
Dallas, Texas

Joseph I. Shapiro, MD
Mercy Health Partners Education Professor
Chairman, Department of Medicine
Associate Dean for Business Development
Professor of Medicine and Pharmacology
The University of Toledo College of Medicine
Toledo, Ohio

Youngsook Yoon, MD
Associate Professor of Medicine
Division of Pulmonary and Critical Care Medicine
Department of Medicine
The University of Toledo College of Medicine
Toledo, Ohio

Preface

An important part of all aspects of internal medicine and nephrology are the areas of electrolyte homeostasis, and acid-base and mineral metabolism. Disturbances of fluid and electrolyte balance, and disorders of acid-base and mineral metabolism homeostasis are often confusing to most trainees and non-nephrology physicians. It is imperative that clinicians early in their training as medical students, physician assistants, house officers, and subspecialty fellows gain a solid understanding of basic aspects of these disorders. This manual was conceived to provide a readily available pocket guide to remove that confusion. *Lange Instant Access: Acid-Base, Fluids, and Electrolytes* provides a comprehensive and concise text for physicians in training and practitioners.

This manual is an ideal tool for health care providers to rapidly attain a complete understanding of the basics of electrolytes and fluid disorders and acid-base and divalent disturbances, allowing an educated approach to diagnosis and management of these disorders. The book will be a handy reference upon which they can build by utilizing other sources of information such as primary literature from journals and more detailed textbooks. It will also serve as an efficient resource for non-nephrology practitioners in internal medicine and other fields of medicine and surgery.

Lange Instant Access: Acid-Base, Fluids, and Electrolytes is broken down into three major sections. The first section discusses electrolyte disorders; the second acid-base disturbances; and the third, mineral metabolism. Hopefully, after reading this book the reader will begin to comprehend the complex world of electrolytes, acid-base, and mineral metabolism.

Acknowledgments

I wish to thank Drs. Peter Igarashi, Peter Aronson, David Ellison, Gary Desir, Asghar Rastegar, Norman Siegel, John Forrest, John Hayslett, Robert Schrier, Allen Alfrey, Laurence Chan, and Tomas Berl, who served as mentors and teachers during my career. I would also like to thank Drs. Gregory Fitz, Clark Gregg, Charles Pak, Orson Moe, and Khashayar Sakhaee for their help in recruiting me to my current position.

Robert F. Reilly, Jr.

I wish to thank Drs. Peter Aronson, Asghar Rastegar, John Hayslett, Peggy Bia, Stefan Somlo, Rex Mahnensmith, Norman Siegel, Michael Kashgarian, Stephen Huot, David Ellison, Robert Piscatelli, Gregory Buller, Majid Sadigh, and K. Jega, who served as mentors and teachers during my career. I would also like to thank my many colleagues in medicine and nephrology, in particular Drs. Ursula Brewster and Richard Sherman, who have been a source of inspiration during my career.

Mark A. Perazella

1

Body Fluid Compartments and Intravenous Fluid Replacement

BODY FLUID COMPARTMENTS

TABLE 1-1: Body Fluid Compartments
An understanding of body fluid compartments is essential to provide adequate patient care and for appropriate and intelligent use of intravenous fluid replacement solutions
TBW constitutes 60% of lean body weight in men, 50% of lean body weight in women
• ICF compartment (two-thirds of TBW)
• ECF fluid compartment (one-third of TBW)
ECF compartment includes
• Intravascular space (25% of ECF)
• Interstitial space (75% of ECF)
Osmotic forces govern water distribution between ICF and ECF (see Figures 1-1 and 1-2)
• Water flows from low osmolality to high osmolality
• Solute addition to the ECF raises osmolality
■ Water flows out of ICF until the gradient is gone
■ Water moves into and out of cells, resulting in cell swelling or shrinking
Abbreviations: TBW, total body water; ECF, extracellular fluid; ICF, intracellular fluid

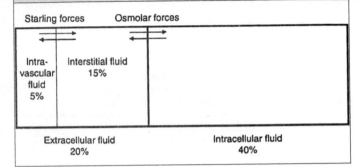

FIGURE 1–1: Body fluids are contained within the intracellular fluid compartment and the extracellular fluid compartment, which is composed of the interstitial and intravascular fluid compartments

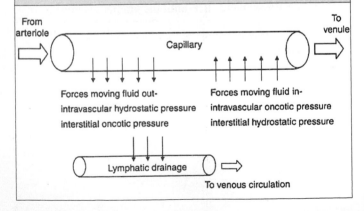

FIGURE 1–2: Factors Influencing Fluid Movement between Various Compartments within the Body. Starling forces govern water movement between intravascular and interstitial spaces. Edema formation occurs from an increase in capillary hydrostatic pressure and/or a decrease in capillary oncotic pressure

TABLE 1–2: Major Water-Retaining Solute in Each Compartment
Extracellular fluid compartment—Na^+ salts
Intracellular fluid compartment—K^+ salts
Intravascular space—plasma proteins

TABLE 1–3: Increased ECF Volume with Variable Serum Na$^+$ Concentration

Serum Na$^+$ concentration [Na$^+$] is a ratio of the amounts of Na$^+$ and water in the ECF

Three examples illustrate increased ECF volume where serum Na$^+$ concentration is high, low, and normal

Addition of NaCl to the ECF

- Na$^+$ remains within the ECF

- Osmolality increases and water moves out of cells

- Equilibrium is characterized by relative *hypernatremia*

- ECF volume increases and ICF volume decreases

- Na$^+$ increases osmolality of both ECF and ICF

Addition of 1 L of water to the ECF

- Osmolality decreases, moving water into cells

- Equilibrium is characterized by relative *hyponatremia*

- Expansion of both ECF and ICF volumes occurs

- Only 80 mL remains in the intravascular space

Addition of 1 L of isotonic saline to the ECF

- Saline remains in the ECF (increases by 1L)

- Intravascular volume increases by 250 mL

- There is no change in osmolality

  - No shift of water between the ECF and ICF

  - Serum Na$^+$ concentration is unchanged

Abbreviations: ECF, extracellular fluid; ICF, intracellular fluid

TABLE 1–4: Mechanism of Edema Formation	
Increased Hydrostatic Pressure	**Decreased Capillary Oncotic Pressure**
Congestive heart failure	Nephrotic syndrome
Cirrhosis of the liver	Cirrhosis of the liver
Venous obstruction	Malabsorption

INTRAVENOUS SOLUTIONS

TABLE 1–5: Critical Elements of IV Solution Use
IV solutions are used to expand intravascular and extracellular fluid spaces
Assessment of the patient's volume status
• Hypovolemia is common in hospitalized patients, especially in critical care units
• Obvious fluid loss (hemorrhage or diarrhea)
• No obvious fluid loss (third spacing from vasodilation with sepsis or anaphylaxis)
Knowledge of available solutions
• Colloid versus crystalloid
• Space of distribution
• Cost and potential adverse effects
Abbreviation: IV, intravenous

TABLE 1–6: Replacement Options: Colloid versus Crystalloid

Crystalloid solutions consist primarily of water and dextrose
Crystalloids rapidly leave the intravascular space and enter the interstitial space
Colloid solutions consist of various osmotically active agents
Colloids remain in the intravascular space longer than crystalloids

TABLE 1–7: Replacement Fluid Options: Crystalloid Solutions

Solution	Osm	Glucose	Na$^+$	Cl$^-$	Lactate
D5W	252	50	—	—	—
0.9% NS	308	—	154	154	—
0.45% NS	154	—	77	77	—
Ringer's lactate	272	—	130	109	28

Abbreviations: Osm, osmolality; D5W, 5% dextrose in water; NS, normal saline

Units: Osm, mOsm/L; glucose, g/L; Na$^+$, Cl$^-$, and lactate, mEq/L

TABLE 1–8: Replacement Fluids: Colloid Solution Characteristics

Colloids increase osmotic pressure and remain in the intravascular space for longer periods
Osmotic pressure is proportional to the number of particles in solution
Colloids do not readily cross normal capillary walls
They promote fluid translocation from interstitial space to intravascular space
Colloids include HES, dextran, and albumin
Colloids characteristics
• Monodisperse (albumin); MW is uniform
• Polydisperse (starches); MWs are in different ranges
Colloid MW determines the duration of colloidal effect in intravascular space
Small MW colloids
• Large initial oncotic effect
• Rapid renal excretion
• Shorter duration of action
Abbreviations: HES, hydroxyethyl starch; MW, molecular weight

TABLE 1–9: HES as a Plasma Volume Expander

HES is a glucose polymer derived from amylopectin

Hydroxyethyl groups are substituted for hydroxyl groups on glucose

HES has a wide MW range (Polydisperse)

- Slower degradation and increased water solubility

- Degraded by circulating amylases and are insoluble at neutral pH

One liter of HES expands the intravascular space by 700–1000 mL

Duration of action depends on rates of elimination and degradation

- Smaller MW species are rapidly excreted by kidney

- Degradation rate is determined by the following:

  - Degree of substitution (the percentage of glucose molecules having a hydroxyethyl group substituted for a hydroxyl group)

  - Location of substitution (positions C2, C3, and C6 of glucose)

Characteristics associated with a longer duration of action

- Large MW

- High degree of substitution and a high C2/C6 ratio

TABLE 1–9 (Continued)
Hetastarch (type of HES) characteristics
• Large MW (670 kDa)
• Slow elimination kinetics
• Increased risk of bleeding complications after cardiac and neurosurgery due to these characteristics
• Increased risk of acute kidney injury in septic and critically ill patients and in brain-dead kidney donors
• HES is contraindicated in the setting of kidney dysfunction
Abbreviations: HES, hydroxyethyl starch; MW, molecular weight

TABLE 1–10: Characteristics of Albumin and Hetastarch		
	Albumin	**Hetastarch**
Molecular weight	69,000	670,000
Made from	Human sera	Starch
Compound	Protein	Amylopectin
Preparations	25% and 5%	6%

TABLE 1–11: Dextran as a Plasma Volume Expander

Dextrans are glucose polymers (MW ≈ 40–70 kDa) with anticoagulant properties

Decrease risk of postoperative deep venous thrombosis and pulmonary embolism

Decrease concentrations of von Willebrand factor and factor VIII:c

Enhance fibrinolysis and protect plasmin from the inhibitory effects of α_2-antiplasmin

Increase blood loss after prostate and hip surgery

Increase acute kidney injury in acute ischemic stroke

Abbreviations: MW, molecular weight

TABLE 1–12: Albumin as a Plasma Volume Expander

Available in two different concentrations

- 5% solution: albumin (12.5 g) in 250 mL of normal saline has a COP of 20 mmHg

- 25% solution: albumin (12.5 g) in 50 mL of normal saline has a COP of 100 mmHg

One liter of 5% albumin expands the intravascular space by 500–1000 mL

Compared with crystalloid, albumin increases mortality risk in certain patient groups, but the data are mixed

Mortality concerns and cost limit albumin use

Abbreviations: COP, colloid osmotic pressure

TABLE 1–13: Adverse Effects of Crystalloids and Colloids

Colloids and crystalloids are not different in rates of pulmonary edema, mortality, or length of hospital stay

Crystalloids

- Excessive expansion of interstitial space

- Predisposition to pulmonary edema

Colloids

- Potential to leak into the interstitial space when capillary walls are damaged

GENERAL PRINCIPLES

TABLE 1–14: General Rules for Correction of the Fluid Deficit

Physical examination and the clinical situation determine the amount of Na^+ and volume required

- Three to five liters in the patient with a history of volume loss

- Five to seven liters in the patient with orthostatic hypotension

- Seven to ten liters in the hypotensive septic patient

TABLE 1–15: Basics of Fluid Choice (Colloid vs. Crystalloid)
Colloids are initially confined to the intravascular space, thus requiring about one-fourth of these volumes
Crystalloids are preferred in bleeding patients
Colloids minimize Na^+ overload in patients with total body salt and water excess (CHF, cirrhosis, nephrosis)
Albumin is used with large volume paracentesis in cirrhotics and in the setting of cardiopulmonary bypass
Crystalloids such as normal saline and Ringer's lactate or colloids are the fluid of choice in hypotensive patients
In patients with identifiable sources of fluid loss knowledge of electrolyte content of body fluids is important
Abbreviation: CHF, congestive heart failure

TABLE 1–16: Electrolyte Content of Body Fluids				
	Na^+ (mEq/L)	K^+ (mEq/L)	Cl^- (mEq/L)	HCO_3^- (mEq/L)
Sweat	30–50	5	50	—
Gastric	40–60	10	100	0
Pancreatic	150	5–10	80	70–80
Duodenum	90	10–20	90	10–20
Ileum	40	10	60	70
Colon	40	90	20	30

TABLE 1–17: Insensible Losses and Maintenance Requirements

Insensible water losses average 500–1000 mL/day or approximately 10 mL/kg/day

Insensible water losses are less in the ventilated patient breathing humidified air and higher in febrile patients

Daily maintenance requirements for Na^+ are 50–100 mEq/day, K^+ are 40–80 mEq/day, and glucose are 150 g/day

ASSESSING EXTRACELLULAR FLUID VOLUME

TABLE 1–18: Assessment of ECF Volume

Symptoms and signs, in particular BP changes, are employed to assess ECF volume

Symptoms

• Thirst, dry mouth, and dizziness

Signs

• Diminished axillary sweat, decreased capillary refill, and poor skin turgor

Orthostatic hypotension is a more reliable physical examination finding of ECF volume depletion

Orthostatic hypotension is defined as the following BP changes

• Decline in systolic BP ≥ 20 mmHg

• Decrease in diastolic BP ≥ 10 mmHg

Abbreviations: ECF, extracellular fluid; BP, blood pressure

FLUID RESUSCITATION

TABLE 1–19: Monitoring Fluid Resuscitation
Fluid resuscitation requires boluses of crystalloid or colloid with close clinical monitoring
Monitor with periodic reassessment of blood pressure, heart rate, and urine output
Patients with advanced chronic kidney disease or end-stage renal disease cannot be monitored by urine output
Patients that do not respond or who have severe heart or lung disease are considered for invasive monitoring
• Central venous pressure and pulmonary artery occlusion pressure measurements are used as gold standard of LV preload
• Cardiac output is optimal at central filling pressures of 12–15 mmHg
Pulmonary artery occlusion pressure and LV end-diastolic pressure are affected by intrathoracic pressure and myocardial compliance with mechanical ventilation
Abbreviation: LV, left ventricular

CLINICAL EXAMPLES OF FLUID RESUSCITATION

TABLE 1–20: The Septic Patient
Cardiac output is generally high and systemic vascular resistance low in septic shock
Tissue perfusion is compromised by both systemic hypotension and maldistribution of blood flow in the microcirculation
Fluid resuscitation aims at normalization of tissue perfusion and oxidative metabolism
• Increased cardiac output and blood and plasma volumes are associated with improved survival
• Fluid resuscitation increases cardiac index by 25–40% and reverses hypotension in as many as 50% of septic patients
• Deficits require 2–4 L of colloid and 5–10 L of crystalloid
Acute respiratory distress syndrome develops in one-third to two-thirds of septic patients
• Beneficial effects of volume expansion on vital organ perfusion are balanced against potential worsening of noncardiogenic pulmonary edema

TABLE 1–21: Crystalloids versus Colloids in the Septic Patient

Both crystalloids and colloids may worsen pulmonary edema
Crystalloids lower plasma oncotic pressure and drive water out of the intravascular space and into the lungs
Colloid particles migrate into the interstitium if microvascular permeability is increased, acting as a driving force for water movement into the lungs
Crystalloids and colloids cause equal rates of pulmonary edema when low filling pressures are maintained

TABLE 1–22: The Cardiac Surgery Patient

Cardiac surgery is associated with risk for intraoperative and postoperative bleeding
Increased post cardiopulmonary bypass blood loss requiring reoperation is an independent risk factor for prolonged intensive care unit stay and death
Cardiopulmonary bypass increases bleeding by inducing multiple platelet abnormalities
• Decreased platelet counts and reduced von Willebrand factor receptors
• Desensitization of platelet thrombin receptors
• Cardiopulmonary bypass activates inflammatory mediators and complement
• Increases free radical generation and lipid peroxidation

TABLE 1–23: Albumin versus Hetastarch in CPB

Trials comparing hetastarch to albumin show increased postoperative bleeding and higher transfusion requirements with hetastarch

- Increased blood loss occurs with hetastarch even in low risk patients

- A 25% lower mortality is noted with albumin versus hetastarch

Albumin is preferred in the setting of CPB due to the following:

- It has antioxidant properties

- Inhibits apoptosis in microvascular endothelium

Albumin coats the surface of the extracorporeal circuit

- Decreases polymer surface affinity for platelets

- Reduces platelet granule release

Hetastarch reduces von Willebrand factor and receptor function

- Promotes platelet dysfunction and increases bleeding risk

Abbreviation: CPB, cardiopulmonary bypass

2

Disorders of Na⁺ Balance
(Edema, Hypertension, or Hypotension)

INTRODUCTION

TABLE 2–1: Basics of Na$^+$ Balance
Disorders of ECF volume are due to disturbances in Na$^+$ balance
ECF volume control depends on regulation of Na$^+$ balance, which reflects the Na$^+$ content of the body
Na$^+$ concentration reflects water balance, not Na$^+$ balance or content. Disorders of Na$^+$ concentration (hypo- and hypernatremia) are due to disturbances in:
• Water balance
• ECF volume
■ Balance between Na$^+$ intake and Na$^+$ excretion
■ Regulated by a complex system acting via the kidney
Normally, Na$^+$ balance is maintained without edema or BP changes across a broad range of Na$^+$ intake (10–1000 mEq/day)
Abbreviations: ECF, extracellular fluid; BP, blood pressure

TABLE 2–2: States of ECF Volume

States where ECF volume is increased

Net gain of total body Na+

Edema and/or hypertension

States where ECF volume is decreased

Total body Na+ deficit

Na+ and water losses from the GI or GU tracts

Decreased blood pressure or shock

Abbreviations: ECF, extracellular fluid; GI, gastrointestinal; GU, genitourinary

TABLE 2–3: Sensors and Effectors of Na+ Balance

Sensors detect changes in Na+ balance (intravascular filling) and effectors respond by adjusting renal Na+ excretion

Na+ Sensors	Effectors
Low pressure receptors (atria/veins)	Glomerular filtration rate
High pressure receptors (aortic arch and carotid sinus)	Peritubular physical factors (ionic, osmotic, and hydraulic gradients)
Hepatic volume receptor	Sympathetic nervous system
Cerebrospinal fluid Na+ receptor	Renin-angiotensin-aldosterone system
Renal afferent arteriole receptors	Atrial natriuretic factor
	Other natriuretic hormones

TABLE 2–4: Interaction of EABV and Renal Na$^+$ Handling
EABV defines the activity of renal Na$^+$ homeostasis effector mechanisms
• It is the relationship between cardiac output and peripheral vascular resistance that is sensed by the high and low pressure baroreceptors
• EABV is a concept not a measured volume
• It estimates net level of stimulation of all Na$^+$ sensors
Renal Na$^+$ retention infers that EABV is decreased
Renal Na$^+$ excretion infers that EABV is increased
Abbreviation: EABV, effective arterial blood volume

REGULATION OF Na$^+$ TRANSPORT IN KIDNEY

TABLE 2–5: Na$^+$ Transport in the Kidney
Based on the state of the ECF volume (EABV), renal Na$^+$ transport responds with either Na$^+$ reabsorption (ECF volume depletion) or Na$^+$ excretion (ECF volume excess)
Decreased ECF volume reduces renal Na$^+$ excretion by (1) decreasing filtered Na$^+$ and (2) increasing tubular Na$^+$ reabsorption; these effects also increase salt and water craving
Increased ECF volume has the opposite effects on renal Na$^+$ handling, salt craving, and thirst
Abbreviations: ECF, extracellular fluid; EABV, effective arterial blood volume

| TABLE 2–6: Systemic Effects of ECF Volume Status ||
ECF Volume Expansion	ECF Volume Depletion
Reduces Na$^+$ and water retention	**Enhances Na$^+$ and water retention**
• Suppresses release of angiotensin II, aldosterone, and arginine vasopressin	• Stimulates release of angiotensin II, aldosterone, and arginine vasopressin
• Inactivates the SNS	• Activates the SNS
Decreases tubular Na$^+$ reabsorption	**Increases tubular Na$^+$ reabsorption**
• Inactivates RAAS, changes peritubular physical forces, and increases natriuretic peptides	• Activates RAAS, changes peritubular physical forces, and suppresses natriuretic peptides
Abolishes thirst and salt craving	**Stimulates thirst and salt craving**
• Low angiotensin II and aldosterone reduce salt appetite	• Angiotensin II and aldosterone stimulate salt appetite
• Low angiotensin II diminishes thirst	• Angiotensin II also stimulates thirst
Abbreviations: ECF, extracellular fluid; SNS, sympathetic nervous system; RAAS, renin-angiotensin-aldosterone system	

Na$^+$ TRANSPORT ALONG THE NEPHRON

Renal Na$^+$ handling occurs along various nephron sites, starting with filtration at the glomerulus and including both reabsorption and secretion by various tubular cells.

TABLE 2–7: Glomerulus (Glomerular Filtration)
Glomerulus freely filters NaCl
Filtered NaCl load is 1.7 kg/day
Filtered NaCl load is eleven times the amount of NaCl that resides in ECF
Less than 1% of filtered Na$^+$ is excreted in urine, which is under the control of effector mechanisms that regulate Na$^+$ reabsorption
Abbreviation: ECF, extracellular fluid

TABLE 2–8: Proximal Tubule
Proximal tubule reabsorbs 60–70% of filtered NaCl load
The principal pathway for Na$^+$ entry is via the Na$^+$-H$^+$ exchanger (NHE3)
Physical factors, the SNS and RAAS, regulate Na$^+$ reabsorption
Physical factors regulate Na$^+$ reabsorption through changes in FF that create hydrostatic and oncotic gradients for water movement
The FF is the ratio of GFR to RPF
• FF = GFR/RPF
Efferent arteriolar constriction by AII increases the FF via the following mechanisms
Reduces renal blood flow (decreases RPF)
Increases glomerular capillary pressure (raises GFR)
Rise in FF increases oncotic pressure and decreases hydrostatic pressure in the peritubular capillary
• This promotes reabsorption of salt and water
The RAAS has direct effects on tubular transport mediated via NHE3 and Na$^+$-K$^+$ ATPase
AII and aldosterone upregulate NHE3
AII stimulates Na$^+$-K$^+$ ATPase enzyme activity
The SNS and insulin stimulate NHE3 activity

(continued)

TABLE 2–8 (Continued)

Systemic BP modifies proximal tubular Na^+ reabsorption; as BP rises, renal excretion of NaCl increases (pressure natriuresis)

Pressure natriuresis is not mediated by an increase in filtered Na^+ load; but is mediated by reduced Na^+ reabsorption

With increased BP the afferent arteriole constricts to maintain glomerular capillary hydrostatic pressure constant

Afferent arteriolar constriction results from

- Direct myogenic reflex

- TGF

Increased BP is sensed in the vasculature; signal is sent to proximal tubule to reduce tubular NaCl reabsorption

- Mediated by removal of NHE3 from the luminal membrane of the proximal tubule

- Na^+-K^+ ATPase activity is also decreased

MD cells sense increased NaCl delivery to the thick ascending limb of Henle

The MD is a specialized region near the junction of the cortical TALH and the distal convoluted tubule

The MD is in proximity to granular renin-producing cells in the afferent arteriole of the JG apparatus

JG apparatus mediates TGF by the following:

- Increased NaCl delivery is sensed by MD, renin release is suppressed and AII levels fall

- Decreased NaCl delivery is sensed by MD, renin release is stimulated and the RAAS activated

TABLE 2–8 (Continued)

TGF serves two purposes

- Short term—maintains constant NaCl delivery to distal nephron segments

- Long term—controls renin secretion to maintain Na⁺ balance

Abbreviations: SNS, sympathetic nervous system; RAAS, renin-angiotensin-aldosterone system; FF, filtration fraction; GFR, glomerular filtration rate; RPF, renal plasma flow; AII, angiotensin II; BP, blood pressure; MD, macula densa; TALH, thick ascending limb of Henle; JG, juxtaglomerular; TGF, tubuloglomerular feedback

TABLE 2–9: Thick Ascending Limb of Henle

The TALH reabsorbs 20–30% of the filtered NaCl load

Na^+ and Cl^- enter the TALH cell via the Na^+-K^+-$2Cl^-$ cotransporter, which is inhibited by loop diuretics

A ROMK channel in the luminal membrane mediates K^+ recycling to allow optimal NaCl reabsorption

NaCl absorption in this segment is load dependent. The higher the delivered NaCl load the higher the absorption

Alpha-adrenergic agonists, arginine vasopressin, parathyroid hormone, calcitonin and glucagon increase Na^+ reabsorption

Prostaglandin E_2 inhibits Na^+ reabsorption in this segment

Abbreviations: TALH, thick ascending limb of Henle; ROMK, rat outer medullary potassium

TABLE 2–10: Distal Convoluted Tubule
The DCT reabsorbs 5–10% of the filtered Na$^+$ load
Na$^+$ and Cl$^-$ enter the DCT cell via the thiazide-sensitive NCC and Na$^+$ exits through the Na$^+$-K$^+$ ATPase
• Aldosterone upregulates NCC expression
• The DCT can be subdivided into two parts: (1) an early DCT1 and (2) late DCT2 segment
• DCT2 contains the aldosterone responsive ENaC
• Type-2 11 β-HSD degrades cortisol to inactive cortisone (prevents glucocorticoid binding to the mineralocorticoid receptor and activation of ENaC)
• Expression studies revealed that the mineralocorticoid receptor has equal affinity for glucocorticoids and mineralocorticoids. Glucocorticoids circulate at much higher concentration than mineralocorticoids. It is type-2 11 β-HSD that ensures a specific mineralocorticoid effect and not the receptor itself
• The mineralocorticoid receptor is expressed in DCT, while type-2 11 β-HSD is expressed in the later part of the DCT—DCT2
• PHA II is an autosomal dominant disease of activated NCC characterized by hypertension, hyperkalemia, and thiazide sensitivity (see Table 6–44)
• Mutations in two members of the WNK—WNK1 and WNK4—cause the disease
Abbreviations: DCT, distal convoluted tubule; NCC, Na$^+$-Cl$^-$ cotransporter; ENaC, epithelial Na$^+$ channel; HSD, hydroxysteroid dehydrogenase; PHA II, Pseudohypoaldosteronism type II; WNK, with no lysine (K) kinase family

TABLE 2–11: Cortical Collecting Duct

CCD reabsorbs 1–3% of filtered Na$^+$ load

- Na$^+$ enters the CCD cell via ENaC and exits through the basolateral Na$^+$-K$^+$ ATPase

- ENaC is composed of three subunits (α, β, δ)

- Aldosterone and AII increase ENaC abundance in CCD

- Liddle's syndrome is an autosomal dominant disorder characterized by early onset hypertension, hypokalemia, and metabolic alkalosis (see Table 7–15)

- Results from mutations in α- and β-ENaC subunits that increase ENaC activity

Abbreviations: CCD, cortical collecting duct; ENaC, epithelial Na$^+$ channel; AII, angiotensin II

TABLE 2–12: Medullary Collecting Duct

In IMCD Na$^+$ enters the cell via ENaC and a cyclic GMP gated cation channel that transports Na$^+$, K$^+$, and NH$_4^+$

The cyclic GMP gated cation channel is inhibited by natriuretic peptides, the major regulator of Na$^+$ transport in IMCD

Abbreviations: IMCD, inner medullary collecting duct; ENaC, epithelial Na$^+$ channel; GMP, guanosine monophosphate

TABLE 2–13: Natriuretic Peptides
Natriuretic peptides are a family of proteins
• ANP
• Long acting atrial natriuretic peptide
• Vessel dilator
• Kaliuretic peptide
• BNP
• CNP
• Urodilatin
Three types of NPR exist
NPR-A and NPR-B are isoforms of guanylate cyclase
NPR-A catalyze the conversion of GTP to cyclic GMP
NPR-B may be a specific receptor for CNP
Atrial natriuretic peptide acts through NPR-A
Sites of natriuretic peptide production
• ANP—cardiac atrium
• BNP—cardiac ventricles
• CNP—endothelial cells
• Urodilatin—distal tubule of kidney
Natriuretic peptides protect against ECF volume expansion, especially in congestive heart failure
Abbreviations: ANP, atrial natriuretic peptide; BNP, brain-type natriuretic peptide; CNP, C-type natriuretic peptide; NPR, natriuretic peptide receptors; GTP, guanosine triphosphate; GMP, guanosine monophosphate; ECF, extracellular fluid

DISORDERS ASSOCIATED WITH INCREASED TOTAL BODY Na$^+$ (ECF VOLUME EXPANSION)

Hypervolemic states (increased ECF volume) are associated with increased total body Na$^+$ and edema that occurs with or without hypertension.

TABLE 2–14: Definition of Edema
Edema is the accumulation of excess interstitial fluid
Expansion of the interstitial space by 3–5 L results in either localized (vascular or lymphatic injury) or generalized (congestive heart failure) edema
Edema is an indentation or "pitting" that results after applying digital pressure on the skin of the lower extremity or sacrum

TABLE 2–15: Pathophysiology of Edema Formation
Increased formation
• Increased capillary hydrostatic pressure
■ Venous/lymphatic obstruction
■ Congestive heart failure
■ Cirrhosis of the liver
■ Increased capillary permeability
Decreased removal
• Decreased plasma colloid osmotic pressure
■ Nephrotic syndrome
■ Malabsorption
■ Cirrhosis of the liver
• Impaired lymphatic outflow
Ill-defined mechanisms
• Idiopathic cyclic edema
• Pregnancy
• Hypothyroidism
Renal retention of excess salt and water maintains edema

TABLE 2–16: Pathophysiology of ECF Volume Expansion States
Hypertension present, edema present
• Kidney disease
Hypertension present, edema absent
• Mineralocorticoid excess
■ Primary aldosteronism
■ Renal artery stenosis
■ Renin-producing tumors
• Glucocorticoids binding to the mineralocorticoid receptor
■ Cushing's disease
■ Licorice ingestion
■ Apparent mineralocorticoid excess
• Genetic diseases associated with increased distal nephron Na$^+$ reabsorption
■ Liddle's syndrome
■ Pseudohypoaldosteronism type II (Gordon's syndrome)
Hypertension absent, edema present
• Decreased cardiac output
■ Congestive heart failure
■ Constrictive pericarditis
■ Pulmonary hypertension

(continued)

TABLE 2–16 (Continued)
• Decreased oncotic pressure
▪ Nephrotic syndrome
• Peripheral vasodilation
▪ Cirrhosis
▪ High-output heart failure
▪ Pregnancy
• Increased capillary permeability
▪ Burns
▪ Sepsis
Abbreviation: ECF, extracellular fluid

CLINICAL MANIFESTATIONS OF INCREASED TOTAL BODY Na$^+$ (ECF VOLUME EXPANSION)

TABLE 2–17: Hypertension Present, Edema Present
Kidney disease and decreased GFR
• Decrease in renal function causes Na$^+$ retention and ECF volume expansion with hypertension and edema
Acute GN results in primary NaCl retention with edema and hypertension
• Acute poststreptococcal GN has low renin activity and increased concentration of atrial natriuretic peptides supporting ECF volume expansion
Abbreviations: GFR, glomerular filtration rate; ECF, extracellular fluid GN, glomerulonephritis

TABLE 2–18: Hypertension Present, Edema Absent

Excess mineralocorticoids promote renal Na$^+$ retention

Disorders of mineralocorticoid excess include primary aldosteronism, renal artery stenosis, and renin-producing tumors

Disorders associated with glucocorticoids binding to the mineralocorticoid receptor include Cushing's syndrome, licorice ingestion, and apparent mineralocorticoid excess

Genetic diseases that increase Na$^+$ reabsorption in distal nephron

- Liddle's syndrome—overactivity of ENaC in the CCD

- PHA II—overactivity of NCC in the DCT

The kidney is able to maintain ECF volume homeostasis but at the cost of hypertension in all of these disorders

The relationship between defects in renal salt excretion and subsequent development of hypertension

- Long-term increases in BP occur due to decreased renal salt and water excretion

- In normals exposed to a salt load

  - Increased arterial pressure enhances Na$^+$ excretion and returns BP to normal, mediated via pressure natriuresis

  - A steady state is reestablished where Na$^+$ intake equals Na$^+$ excretion at a normal BP

  - Increased salt intake transiently raises BP (Figure 2–1—arrow #1); pressure natriuresis returns BP to normal (Figure 2–1—arrow #2)

  - Pressure natriuresis stabilizes BP and ECF volume

(continued)

TABLE 2–18 (Continued)

- Diseases that increase preglomerular resistance, increase tubular reabsorption of Na^+, or reduce the number of nephrons cause rightward shifts of the curve (Figure 2–1—activated RAAS curve)

- Since renin is suppressed, renal salt excretion is impaired and requires a higher BP

  - This explains the "salt-sensitive" nature of hypertension in patients with kidney disease

- Renal arteriolar vasodilation and increased single nephron GFR damage surviving nephrons

  - Damage to surviving nephrons shifts the pressure natriuresis curve to the right

Abbreviations: ENaC, epithelial Na^+ channel; CCD, cortical collecting duct; PHA II, Pseudohypoaldosteronism type II; NCC, Na^+-Cl^- cotransporter; DCT, distal convoluted tubule; ECF, extracellular fluid; BP, blood pressure; RAAS, renin-angiotensin-aldosterone system; GFR, glomerular filtration rate

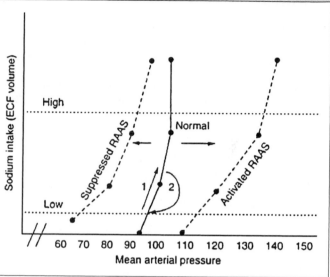

FIGURE 2–1: Interactions between Sodium Intake and Mean Arterial Pressure and the Effect of Various Factors in the Development of Hypertension

TABLE 2–19: Hypertension Absent, Edema Present

CHF, hepatic cirrhosis and nephrotic syndrome are characterized by edema without hypertension

In these disorders a primary abnormality decreases EABV that stimulates effector mechanisms and renal Na$^+$ retention

In CHF, cardiac output is decreased, plasma volume expanded, and a secondary increase in PVR maintains BP

- Arterial underfilling is sensed by baroreceptors

- Effector systems are activated by

  - SNS and RAAS stimulation

  - AVP release (nonosmotic)

- The net effect of increased SNS, AVP, and RAAS activation is salt and water retention

- The intensity of the neurohumoral response is proportional to the severity of the CHF

  - Na$^+$ concentration correlates with AVP concentration

  - Severity of hyponatremia predicts cardiovascular mortality

- Although ANP concentrations are elevated, there is resistance to their action due to increased Na$^+$ reabsorption in nephron segments upstream of the IMCD

In hepatic cirrhosis, PVR is low, which causes a secondary increase in cardiac output

- Plasma volume is increased prior to development of ascites

TABLE 2–19 (Continued)
• Splanchnic vasodilation occurs due to nitric oxide synthesis
▪ Splanchnic vasodilation occurs early and results in arterial underfilling and activation of neurohumoral mechanisms that lead to salt and water retention
• There is a direct correlation between the degree of decrease in PVR and increase in plasma volume
▪ Severity of hyponatremia is predictive of mortality
In nephrotic syndrome, two hypotheses exist to explain edema formation
• Underfill hypothesis and overflow hypothesis
Abbreviations: CHF, congestive heart failure; EABV, effective arterial blood volume; BP, blood pressure; SNS, sympathetic nervous system; RAAS, renin-angiotensin-aldosterone system; AVP, arginine vasopressin; ANP, atrial natriuretic peptide; IMCD, inner medullary collecting duct; PVR, peripheral vascular resistance

TABLE 2–20: Hypotheses for Edema Formation with Nephrotic Syndrome

Underfill hypothesis

- Edema forms as a result of decreased EABV, which is secondary to decreased capillary oncotic pressure that results from hypoalbuminemia

- Reduced oncotic pressure increases fluid movement into the interstitium and reduces ECF volume

- Effector mechanisms are activated increasing renal salt and water reabsorption that maintain the edema

Overflow hypothesis

- Edema is due to a primary increase in renal Na$^+$ reabsorption (like acute glomerulonephritis)

- Expansion of ECF volume and suppression of the RAAS with edema formation occurs

Abbreviations: EABV, effective arterial blood volume; ECF, extracellular fluid; RAAS, renin-angiotensin-aldosterone system

TABLE 2–21: Counterregulatory Hormones in Nephrotic Syndrome

One-half of nephrotic patients have elevated plasma renin activity (underfill subgroup)

Plasma and urinary catecholamine concentrations are often increased (underfill hypothesis)

Plasma AVP concentrations correlate with blood volume and are reduced by albumin infusion (underfill subgroup)

Natriuresis precedes the increase in serum albumin concentration in corticosteroid treated patients with minimal change disease

RAAS activity is commonly suppressed

In animal models of unilateral nephrosis, Na$^+$ is retained in the affected kidney arguing for primary defect in Na$^+$ reabsorption supporting the overflow hypothesis

Subgroups of patients with nephrotic syndrome exist

- Underfilled nephrotic patients will have decreased EABV, activation of RAAS and lack hypertension

- Overflow nephrotic patients demonstrate hypertension, RAAS suppression and a lower GFR

- Overflow patients respond well to diuretics

- Underfilled patients will develop prerenal azotemia with diuretics

Abbreviations: AVP, arginine vasopressin; RAAS, renin-angiotensin-aldosterone system; EABV, effective arterial blood volume; GFR, glomerular filtration rate

TABLE 2–22: Edema without Hypertension from Capillary Leak

Burns can result in localized or generalized edema

- Thermal injury and vasoactive substances cause local edema via capillary vasodilation and increased permeability

- Diffuse edema occurs when full thickness burns involve more than 30% of body surface area

- Reduced capillary oncotic pressure from plasma protein loss into wounds promotes edema

Septic patients with SIRS may develop edema

- Increases in capillary permeability and precapillary vasodilation raise capillary hydrostatic pressure, which increases interstitial oncotic pressure resulting in edema

- Large amounts of intravenous fluids (administered to maintain BP) may worsen edema

- Positive pressure ventilation and positive end expiratory pressure ventilation worsen edema by

  - Reducing cardiac output, which activates the SNS and RAAS (increases renal salt and water reabsorption)

  - Increasing intrathoracic pressure impeding lymphatic drainage through the thoracic duct

Abbreviations: SIRS, severe inflammatory response syndrome; BP, blood pressure; SNS, sympathetic nervous system; RAAS, renin-angiotensin-aldosterone system

GENERAL APPROACH TO THE EDEMATOUS PATIENT

TABLE 2–23: General Approach to the Edematous Patient
Edema is classified as generalized (CHF, cirrhosis) or localized (vascular or lymphatic injury)
Evaluate the patient for evidence of heart, liver, or kidney disease is the next step
Location of edema narrows the differential diagnosis
• Pulmonary edema and an S3 gallop point to left-sided CHF
• Right-sided CHF and cirrhosis of the liver result in edema in the lower extremities or abdomen (ascites)
• Palmar erythema, spider angiomas, hepatomegaly, and caput medusae implicate the liver
Important laboratory studies
• Serum BUN and creatinine concentrations, liver function tests, serum albumin concentration, urinalysis for protein excretion, chest radiograph, and electrocardiogram
Abbreviations: CHF, congestive heart failure; BUN, blood urea nitrogen

GENERAL TREATMENT OF THE EDEMATOUS PATIENT

TABLE 2–24: General Treatment of the Edematous Patient
Reversal of underlying pathophysiology (ACE-inhibitors in CHF) should be utilized when possible
A low salt diet is critical to the success of any regimen
If these measures are unsuccessful a diuretic may be required
Abbreviations: ACE, angiotensin converting enzyme; CHF, congestive heart failure

CLINICAL MANIFESTATIONS OF DECREASED TOTAL BODY Na$^+$ (ECF VOLUME DEPLETION)

TABLE 2–25: Decreased Total Body Na$^+$
Na$^+$ depletion means ECF volume depletion
Na$^+$ depletion does not imply hyponatremia or vice versa
When Na$^+$ excretion exceeds input negative Na$^+$ balance and decreased ECF volume result
Since the normal kidney can lower Na$^+$ excretion to near zero, decreased Na$^+$ intake alone never causes decreased ECF volume
Abbreviation: ECF, extracellular fluid volume

TABLE 2–26: Manifestations of Na$^+$ Depletion	
Symptoms	**Signs**
Increased thirst	Orthostatic fall in blood pressure
Weakness and apathy	Orthostatic rise in pulse
Headache	Decreased pulse volume
Muscle cramps	Decreased jugular venous pressure
Anorexia	Dry skin and decreased sweat
Nausea	Dry mucous membranes
Vomiting	Decreased skin turgor

TABLE 2–27: Sources of Na$^+$ Loss

Na$^+$ depletion results from Na$^+$ losses from three major sources: kidney (salt wasting), skin (excessive sweat), or the GI tract (vomiting, diarrhea)

Renal Na$^+$ losses (Na$^+$ wasting) are due to either intrinsic kidney disease or external influences on renal function

- **Renal diseases:** CKD, nonoliguric AKI, the diuretic phase of AKI, and "salt wasting nephropathy." Salt wasting nephropathy occurs with interstitial nephritis, medullary cystic or polycystic kidney disease, and postobstruction. Patients with "salt wasting nephropathy" have reduced GFR (Stage 3–5 CKD)

- **External factors:** solute diuresis from sodium bicarbonate, glucose, urea, and mannitol; diuretic administration; and mineralocorticoid deficiency

- Renal Na$^+$ loss has urine Na$^+$ concentration >20 mEq/L

Gastrointestinal losses are external or internal

- External losses occur with diarrhea, vomiting, GI suction, or external fistulas

- Internal losses or so-called "third spacing" result from peritonitis, pancreatitis, and small bowel obstruction

- GI losses manifest urine Na$^+$ concentration <20 mEq/L

Skin losses also are external or internal

- Excessive sweating, burns, cystic fibrosis, and adrenal insufficiency

- Skin losses manifest urine Na$^+$ concentration <20 mEq/L

Abbreviations: GI, gastrointestinal; CKD, chronic kidney disease; AKI, acute kidney injury; GFR, glomerular filtration rate

GENERAL APPROACH TO THE VOLUME DEPLETED PATIENT

TABLE 2–28: Approach to the Patient with Decreased ECF Volume
• Identify sources of Na$^+$ loss such as polydipsia, diuretic use, diarrhea, vomiting, and sweating
• Examine for ECF volume contraction (postural BP and pulse changes, hypotension), as well its cause
• Examine for ECF volume contraction (postural BP and pulse changes, hypotension), as well its cause
• Decreased urine Na$^+$ concentration, concentrated urine, BUN to creatinine ratio >20:1, and FENa <1% suggests extrarenal Na$^+$ losses $$\text{FENa} = (U_{Na}/P_{Na}) \div (U_{Cr}/P_{Cr}) \times 100$$
• Na$^+$ losses (diuretics) are associated with FENa <1% (after diuretic dissipated)
• FENa >2% suggests primary renal Na$^+$ loss
• With diuretic therapy, use FEUrea
• FEUrea <35% suggests an extrarenal Na$^+$ loss $$\text{FEUrea} = (U_{Urea}/P_{Urea}) \div (U_{Cr}/P_{Cr}) \times 100$$
Abbreviations: ECF, extracellular fluid; BP, blood pressure; BUN, blood urea nitrogen; FENa, fractional excretion of sodium; FEUrea, fractional excretion of urea

GENERAL TREATMENT OF THE VOLUME DEPLETED PATIENT

TABLE 2–29: Treatment of the Patient with Decreased ECF Volume

- In mild depletion states, treatment of underlying disorder and replacement of dietary salt, and water intake corrects deficits

- When BP and tissue perfusion are compromised, IV fluids are often required

Abbreviations: ECF, extracellular fluid; BP, blood pressure; IV, intravenous

---

TABLE 2–30: Amount and Rate of Repletion Based on Clinical Situation

- Cerebral perfusion and urine output are markers of tissue perfusion

- Postural BP and pulse changes are adequate noninvasive indicators of ECF volume status

- The response to rapid infusion of normal saline or direct measures of cardiovascular pressures is also used

Abbreviations: BP, blood pressure; ECF, extracellular fluid

TABLE 2–31: Choices of ECF Volume Expanders

Fresh frozen plasma and packed red cells are effective as initial intravascular volume expanders (remain in intravascular space)

- Cost and infectious complications limit their use

Isotonic NaCl (normal saline) is an effective volume expander

- Confined to the ECF

- Low cost, availability and lack of infectious complications support its use

Five-percent dextrose in water is a poor intravascular volume expander, as water is distributed in total body water

- Only 8% of the administered volume remains within the intravascular space

Other electrolyte deficiencies may also need to be corrected

- K$^+$ losses occur with diarrhea or vomiting

- Mg^{2+} deficiency may develop with thiazide diuretics and diarrheal illnesses

Abbreviation: ECF, extracellular fluid

3
Disorders of Water Balance
(Hypo- and Hypernatremia)

INTRODUCTION

TABLE 3–1: Serum Na^+ Concentration: Na^+/Water Ratio in ECF
The Na^+ concentration in serum reflects water balance in the body, not Na^+ content
Disorders of water balance account for the vast majority of hypo- and hypernatremia
Serum Na^+ is a concentration term and reflects only the relative amounts of Na^+ and water present in the sample
Serum Na^+ concentration = ECF Na^+/ECF H_2O
Hyponatremia results from either a decrease in the numerator or an increase in the denominator
Hypernatremia results from either an increase in the numerator or a decrease in the denominator
Abbreviation: ECF, extracellular fluid

TABLE 3–2: Regulation of Water Homeostasis
Intact thirst mechanism
Intact AVP release and response
Appropriate renal handling of water
Abbreviation: AVP, arginine vasopressin

TABLE 3–3: Renal and Thirst Mechanisms in Water Homeostasis

Renal free water excretion primarily controls water metabolism, which is regulated by AVP

- Above a P_{osm} of 283, AVP increases by 0.38 pg/mL per 1 mOsm/kg increase in P_{osm}

- U_{osm} is determined by AVP. A rise in AVP of 1 pg/mL increases U_{osm} about 225 mOsm/kg

The two major afferent stimuli for thirst are an increase in plasma osmolality and a decrease in ECF volume

- Thirst is sensed at a plasma osmolality of 294 mOsm/kg

- AVP is maximally stimulated (>5 pg/mL) at this osmolality and is sufficient to fully concentrate the urine

- Arginine vasopressin and AII directly stimulate thirst

Abbreviations: AVP, arginine vasopressin; P_{osm}, plasma osmolality; U_{osm}, urine osmolality; ECF, extracellular fluid; AII, angiotensin II

TABLE 3–4: Osmolality versus Tonicity of a Solution
Osmolality is defined as the number of osmoles of solute divided by the number of kilograms of solvent (independent of a membrane)
Tonicity or "effective osmolality" equals the sum of concentration of solutes and exerts an osmotic force across a membrane
Tonicity is less than osmolality by the total concentration of "ineffective solutes" that it contains
Solutes that are freely permeable across cell membranes such as urea are "ineffective osmoles" (not tonic)
Tonicity determines the net osmolar gradient across the cell membrane that in turn drives water movement
Since Na^+ is the most abundant cation in ECF, its concentration is the major determinant of tonicity and osmolality
• Water moves freely across cell membranes allowing maintenance of osmotic equilibrium between various compartments
Abbreviation: ECF, extracellular fluid

TABLE 3–5: Calculation of Plasma Osmolality

P_{osm} is calculated from the following formula
$$\mathbf{P_{osm}} = 2[Na^+]\ (mEq/L) + [BUN]\ (mg/dL)/2.8 + [Glucose]\ (mg/dL)/18$$

Calculation of tonicity includes Na^+ and glucose. Freezing point depression or vapor pressure techniques measure it directly

Body tonicity, measured as plasma osmolality, is maintained within a narrow range (285–295 mOsm/kg)

Disturbances in body tonicity are reflected by alterations in serum Na^+ concentration and present as hypo- or hypernatremia

Abbreviation: P_{osm}, plasma osmolality

HYPONATREMIA

TABLE 3–6: Basics of Hyponatremia
Hyponatremia (serum Na^+ concentration < 135 mEq/L) is the most frequent electrolyte abnormality (10–15% of hospitalized patients)
Free water intake must exceed free water excretion
Excess water intake with normal renal function
• Hyponatremia due to excessive water intake is rarely observed (psychotic patients that drink from faucets)
• With normal renal function, excessive water intake alone does not cause hyponatremia unless it exceeds about 1 L/h
• Patients with psychogenic polydipsia often have some degree of renal impairment
Continued solute-free water intake with a decreased renal capacity for solute-free water excretion
• The most common mechanism

TABLE 3–7: Essentials of Renal Free Water Excretion

Normal delivery of tubular fluid to distal diluting segments

- Adequate GFR without excessive proximal tubular reabsorption is required to deliver tubular fluid to the diluting segments of kidney (TALH and DCT)

- In volume depletion proximal tubular reabsorption increases and limits the volume of dilute urine excreted

Normal function of the diluting segments

- Fluid is diluted in the water-impermeable TALH and DCT by reabsorption of NaCl

- Na^+ is transported on the Na^+-K^+-$2Cl^-$ cotransporter in TALH and the thiazide-sensitive NCC transporter in DCT

- In the diluting segments, U_{osm} declines to less than P_{osm}, generating free water

Absence of AVP

- AVP suppression prevents solute-free water reabsorption in collecting duct

- This is important since the renal interstitium remains slightly hypertonic even during a water diuresis

- AVP is a nonapeptide produced by neurons in the supraoptic and paraventricular nuclei of the hypothalamus

TABLE 3–7 (Continued)
• The neurons cross the pituitary stalk and terminate in the posterior pituitary, releasing AVP into blood
▪ AVP binds to its receptor (V2) in the basolateral membrane of collecting duct
▪ This activates adenylate cyclase, generates cyclic AMP and inserts water channels (aquaporins-AQP2) into apical membrane increasing water permeability
Adequate solute intake
• In rare circumstances inadequate solute intake can compromise renal free water excretion
▪ Beer drinker's potomania
▪ Tea and toast diet
Abbreviations: GFR, glomerular filtration; TALH, thick ascending limb of Henle; DCT, distal convoluted tubule; NCC, Na^+-Cl^- cotransporter; U_{osm}, urine osmolality; P_{osm}, plasma osmolality; AVP, arginine vasopressin; AMP, adenosine monophosphate

TABLE 3–8: Effect of Solute Intake on Water Homeostasis
The kidney generates large volumes of free water but cannot excrete pure water
The lowest U_{osm} attainable in humans is 50 mOsm/kg
The kidney eliminates the dietary osmolar load (approximately 10 mOsm/kg)
Urine volume required to excrete an osmolar load is
• **Urine volume** = osmolar intake or excretion/U_{osm}
Low solute intake, as in beer drinker's potomania, promotes hyponatremia despite maximally dilute urine
• Example: Solute intake of 150 mOsm/day with a U_{osm} of 50 mOsm/kg produces a urine volume of only 3 L/day (low urine volume limits free water clearance)
• Water intake (> 3 L) could exceed renal free water excretion and cause hyponatremia
Abbreviation: U_{osm}, urine osmolality

TABLE 3–9: AVP is Released by Both Osmotic and Nonosmotic Stimuli

Osmotic stimuli

- A 1% increase in ECF osmolality stimulates AVP release (linear relationship as seen in Figure 3–1)

Nonosmotic stimuli

- Changes in autonomic neural tone such as physical pain, stress, and hypoxia

- Decreases in effective circulating volume

  - Volume depletion causes hyponatremia because nonosmotic stimuli for AVP release predominate over osmotic stimuli

  - AVP has a pressor effect mediated via the V1 receptor, contributing 10% to MAP during volume depletion

  - A 5–10% decrement in blood volume stimulates AVP release (see Figure 3–1)

Abbreviations: ECF, extracellular fluid; AVP, arginine vasopressin; MAP, mean arterial pressure

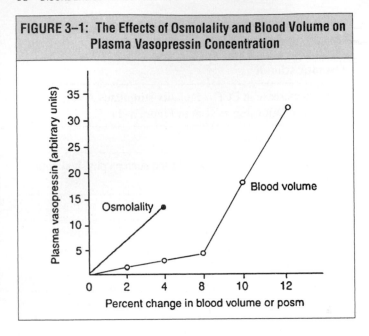

FIGURE 3–1: The Effects of Osmolality and Blood Volume on Plasma Vasopressin Concentration

ETIOLOGY OF HYPONATREMIA

TABLE 3–10: General Categories of Hyponatremia
Hyponatremia may occur in the setting of high, normal, or low serum osmolality
Initial classification of hyponatremia places it into three general categories
• Pseudohyponatremia (normal serum osmolality)
• Translocational hyponatremia (increased serum osmolality)
• True hyponatremia (decreased serum osmolality)

TABLE 3–11: Pseudohyponatremia

An artifactual lowering of Na^+ concentration that is dependent on the method used for measurement

Associated with normal serum osmolality

Plasma is made up of two fractions, aqueous fraction, and particulate fraction

- Pseudohyponatremia results from a decrease in the aqueous fraction

Conditions that reduce the aqueous fraction below the usual 93% of plasma decrease total amount of Na^+ per aliquot of plasma

- Na^+ concentration, however, in the aqueous fraction is normal

Three conditions reduce the aqueous fraction

- Hyperlipidemia and hypercholesterolemia

  ▪ Each 460 mg/dL increase in triglyceride level lowers serum Na^+ concentration by 1 mEq/L

- Hyperproteinemia

  ▪ Excess production of paraproteins (multiple myeloma) increases the particulate fraction

Measurement of serum Na^+ concentration by ion-sensitive electrode yields a normal value provided the sample is not diluted (direct potentiometry); if the sample is diluted (indirect potentiometry) the error is reintroduced. It is key to know the method used in your local laboratory

TABLE 3–12: Translocational Hyponatremia

Shift of water out of cells by a non-Na$^+$ solute; serum osmolality is elevated

Water moves from ICF to ECF when non-Na$^+$ solute increases ECF osmolality

- Hyperglycemia

  - Each increase in serum glucose of 100 mg/dL above normal decreases serum Na$^+$ concentration by 1.6 mEq/L

  - At concentrations greater than 400 mg/dL the correction factor is likely higher (2.4–2.8 mEq/L)

- Mannitol and glycine infusion

  - For each 100 mg/dL rise in glycine concentration, the serum Na$^+$ concentration falls by 3.8 mEq/L

Abbreviations: ICF, intracellular fluid; ECF, extracellular fluid

TABLE 3–13: True Hyponatremia

Associated with a low serum osmolality

Mechanisms

- Excess water intake with normal renal function

- Continued solute-free water intake with a decreased renal capacity for solute-free water excretion

The most common pathophysiologic mechanism is non-osmotic AVP release preventing maximal urinary dilution

The cause of the increased AVP concentration is determined by the patient's volume status

Common causes are edematous states, extrarenal and renal Na^+ and water losses, syndrome of inappropriate ADH (SIADH), and psychogenic polydipsia

Abbreviations: AVP, arginine vasopressin; SIADH, syndrome of inappropriate antidiuretic hormone

TABLE 3–14: True Hyponatremia with Increased ECF Volume

Edema is indicative of increased total body Na^+

Hyponatremia with increased total body Na^+ includes nephrotic syndrome, CHF, hepatic cirrhosis, and acute kidney injury

- Hyponatremia results because the increase in TBW exceeds the increase in total body Na^+

- Effective circulating volume is decreased and stimulation of volume and/or pressure receptors results in AVP release

Abbreviations: ECF, extracellular fluid; CHF, congestive heart failure; TBW, total body water; AVP, arginine vasopressin

TABLE 3–15: True Hyponatremia with Decreased ECF Volume

Renal and extrarenal salt/water losses are characterized by decreased ECF volume resulting in increased thirst, orthostatic hypotension, tachycardia, and decreased skin turgor

- Loss of total body Na^+ exceeds loss of TBW

- AVP release is "appropriate" to defend ECF volume

- With extrarenal fluid loss the Na^+ concentration of the lost fluid is less than serum; hyponatremia develops because thirst is intact and replacement fluid is hypotonic

- Common etiologies of hyponatremia with decreased ECF volume include:

  - GI losses, third spacing of fluids, diuretic overuse or abuse, salt-losing nephritis, adrenal insufficiency, and osmotic diuresis

  - Mineralocorticoid and glucocorticoid deficient states cause volume depletion with nonosmotic AVP release

- Hyponatremia from diuretics

  - Thiazides interfere with urinary dilution but not urinary concentrating ability

  - Thiazide diuretic-induced volume depletion decreases GFR and increases proximal tubular salt and water reabsorption, decreasing water delivery to distal segments, volume contraction also stimulates AVP release

TABLE 3–15 (Continued)

- K^+ depletion results in intracellular shifts of Na^+, and alters sensitivity of the osmoreceptor mechanism leading to AVP release

- Older women are at highest risk

- Loop diuretics interfere with both diluting and concentrating ability, and are associated with less AVP-induced free water reabsorption and much less potential for hyponatremia

Abbreviations: ECF, extracellular fluid; TBW, total body water; AVP, arginine vasopressin; GI, gastrointestinal; GFR, glomerular filtration rate

TABLE 3–16: True Hyponatremia with Clinically Normal ECF Volume

Hyponatremia with clinically normal ECF volume is the result of SIADH or psychogenic polydipsia

- SIADH

  - Though "clinically normal," TBW is increased from "inappropriate" release of AVP

  - "Inappropriate" implies that AVP is released despite the absence of (1) increased serum osmolality and (2) decreased effective circulating volume

  - Mild volume expansion results in urinary Na^+ wasting and clinically undetectable decrease in total body Na^+

  - SIADH is characterized by hyponatremia, low serum osmolality, and inappropriately concentrated urine

  - The urine Na^+ concentration is generally increased but can be low with ECF volume contraction

  - Diagnosis requires clinical euvolemia with no adrenal, renal, or thyroid dysfunction or use of a drug that stimulates AVP release or action

Hyponatremia with clinically normal ECF volume results very rarely from a mutation in the vasopressin V2 receptor gene (R137C or R137L), causing constitutive activation of the V2 receptor and suppressed AVP levels (nephrogenic syndrome of inappropriate antidiuresis)

- Two cases described in male infants with severe hyponatremia

- Novel gain of function mutation in the AVP signaling pathway

Abbreviations: ECF, extracellular fluid; SIADH, syndrome of inappropriate antidiuretic hormone; AVP, arginine vasopressin

TABLE 3–17: Disease Processes Causing SIADH		
Carcinomas	Pulmonary Diseases	CNS Disorders
Lung (small cell)	Viral pneumonia	Encephalitis
Duodenum	Bacterial pneumonia	Meningitis
Pancreas	Pulmonary abscess	Acute psychosis
	Aspergillosis	Porphyria (AIP)
	Mechanical ventilation	Tumors
		Abscesses
		Subdural injury
		Guillain-Barré
		Head trauma
		Stroke

Abbreviations: SIADH, syndrome of inappropriate antidiuretic hormone; CNS, central nervous system; AIP, acute intermittent porphyria

TABLE 3–18: Drugs That Result in AVP Release

Stimulate AVP Release	Other Mechanisms
Nicotine	Chlorpropamide
Clofibrate	Tolbutamide
Vincristine	Cyclophosphamide
Isoproterenol	Morphine
Chlorpropamide	Barbiturates
Antidepressants (SSRIs)	Carbamazepine
Antipsychotic agents	Acetaminophen
Ecstacy	NSAIDs
Amiodarone loading	

Abbreviations: AVP, arginine vasopressin; SSRIs, selective serotonin reuptake inhibitors; NSAIDs, nonsteroidal anti-inflammatory drugs

TABLE 3–19: Other Causes of Euvolemic Hyponatremia

Hypothyroidism impairs renal free water excretion by decreasing GFR, increasing proximal tubular reabsorption, and increasing AVP secretion

Secondary adrenal insufficiency promotes hyponatremia due to nonsuppressed AVP release

Psychogenic polydipsia (water intoxication) results from excess water intake with normal renal function

Abbreviations: GFR, glomerular filtration rate; AVP, arginine vasopressin

SIGNS AND SYMPTOMS

TABLE 3–20: Signs and symptoms of Hyponatremia

Symptom severity correlates both with the magnitude and rapidity of the fall in serum Na^+ concentration

- Gastrointestinal complaints include anorexia, nausea, and vomiting

- Headaches, muscle cramps, and weakness also occur early

- Altered sensorium with impaired response to verbal and painful stimuli, inappropriate behavior, auditory and visual hallucinations, asterixis and obtundation can be seen

- Severe or acute hyponatremia

  - Seizures, or decorticate/decerebrate posturing develop

  - Bradycardia and hyper- or hypotension can occur

  - Respiratory arrest and coma may result

- Central nervous system pathology is due to cerebral edema and symptoms result from a failure in cerebral adaptation

  - When plasma osmolality falls acutely, osmotic equilibrium is maintained by

    - Extrusion of intracellular solutes
    - Influx of water into brain

  - Neurologic symptoms result when osmotic equilibrium is achieved by water influx into brain cells

  - If solute extrusion is successful and osmotic equilibrium maintained, cell swelling is minimized

  - Na^+ extrusion from the brain by Na^+-K^+ ATPase and Na^+ channels is the first pathway activated (minutes)

  - Persistent hyperosmolality activates K^+ channels, which lead to K^+ extrusion (hours)

TABLE 3–21: Neurologic Injury from Hyponatremia

Neurologic injury from hyponatremia is secondary to either hyponatremic encephalopathy or improper therapy (too rapid or overcorrection)

Greater than 90% of cases of neurologic injury are secondary to hyponatremic encephalopathy

Hypoxia is the major factor causing neurologic injury

- Blunts RVD, an ATP-dependent active ion transport process, which allows Na^+ accumulation in the brain and cerebral edema

- Major stimulus for AVP secretion enhancing water entry into neurons

Respiratory arrest and seizures occur suddenly in hyponatremic encephalopathy and are associated with permanent neurologic injury

- Predictive factors include young age, premenopausal state, female sex, and encephalopathy; hypoxia as a result of respiratory arrest or seizure reduces RVD, which in turn exacerbates cerebral edema and often induces permanent neurologic injury

Premenopausal women are at 25-fold increased risk for permanent neurologic injury

- RVD may be decreased in young women (estrogen and progesterone inhibit brain Na^+-K^+ ATPase)

- AVP concentration is higher in women and AVP decreases brain ATP in women but not men

TABLE 3–21: (Continued)
Chronic hyponatremia is characterized by fewer and milder neurologic symptoms
• Regulatory mechanisms promote organic osmolyte (glutamate, taurine, and myoinositol) loss from brain
Abbreviations: RVD, regulatory volume decrease; ATP, adenosine triphosphate; AVP, arginine vasopressin

DIAGNOSIS

TABLE 3–22: Step 1 What Is the Serum Osmolality?
A stepwise approach to hyponatremia ensures accurate diagnosis
Initial evaluation divides the disorder into three broad categories
Iso-osmolar or **pseudohyponatremia**
• Aqueous fraction of plasma is decreased and particulate fraction increased
• Occurs with hyperlipidemia (TG > 1500 mg/dL), hypercholesterolemia or hyperproteinemia
Hyperosmolar or **translocational hyponatremia**
• Due to glucose, mannitol, or glycine
Hypoosmolar or **true hyponatremia**
• Makes up the vast majority of cases
• Divided further based on ECF volume (increased, decreased, or apparently clinically normal)
Abbreviations: TG, triglycerides; ECF, extracellular fluid

TABLE 3–23: Step 2 What is the ECF Volume (Total Body Na$^+$ Content)? Is Dependent Edema Present?

The apparent status of the ECF volume is next addressed; an approach to true hyponatremia is shown in Figure 3–2
Examine the patient for the presence of dependent edema
States of increased ECF volume are characterized by the presence of edema in diseases such as CHF, cirrhosis, nephrotic syndrome, and kidney disease
Abbreviations: ECF, extracellular fluid volume; CHF, congestive heart failure

FIGURE 3–2: Hyponatremia is classified initially based on ECF volume (Total body Na$^+$ content)

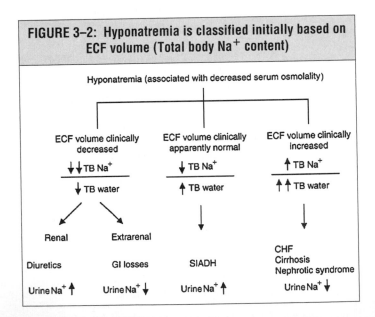

TABLE 3–24: Step 3 What Is the Urine Na$^+$ Concentration?

Absence of edema suggests that the patient's ECF volume is decreased or apparently normal

States of severe ECF volume contraction are clinically apparent while milder degrees are difficult to distinguish from euvolemia (Urine Na$^+$ concentration is useful)

Urine Na$^+$ concentration

- Urine Na$^+$ concentration < 20 mEq/L, U$_{osm}$ > 400 mOsm/kg, and FENa < 1% suggests decreased ECF volume from extrarenal Na$^+$ loss

- Urine Na$^+$ concentration > 20 mEq/L, U$_{osm}$ < 400 mOsm/kg, and FENa > 2% suggests renal Na$^+$ loss

- In the euvolemic patient, consider SIADH, drugs, psychogenic polydipsia, low solute intake, and hypothyroidism

Abbreviations: ECF, extracellular fluid volume; U$_{osm}$, urine osmolality; FENa, fractional excretion of sodium

TREATMENT

TABLE 3–25: Treatment of Hyponatremia
Appropriate treatment depends on the acuity and severity of hyponatremia and ECF volume status
The serum Na^+ concentration is corrected slowly to avoid central pontine myelinolysis if hyponatremia developed over greater than 48 h or the duration is unknown; more rapid correction is appropriate if the hyponatremia developed over < 48 h
Destruction occurs in myelin sheaths of pontine neurons
• Oligodendrocytes in the pons are susceptible to osmotic stress from excessive neuronal dehydration
• Flaccid quadriplegia, dysarthria, dysphagia, coma, and death result
Demyelination can occur with the following:
• Increases in serum $[Na^+]$ to normal within 24–48 h
• Increases in serum $[Na^+]$ greater than 25 mEq/L in the first 48 h
• Increases in serum $[Na^+]$ to hypernatremic levels in patients with liver disease with or without hypokalemia
In states of over-rapid correction, dD-AVP (1-deamino-8-D-arginine vasopressin) may slow or reverse the rate of rise of serum $[Na^+]$
• The risk of re-lowering serum $[Na^+]$ is probably low in the first few days of correction
• As serum $[Na^+]$ rises during the correction phase, the brain regains extruded osmolytes (completed within 5–7 days)
Abbreviation: ECF, extracellular fluid volume

TABLE 3–26: Treatment of Severe, Symptomatic Hyponatremia

Severe symptomatic hyponatremia ($\pm$ seizures) is treated emergently to raise serum Na^+ concentration above 120 mEq/L

Symptomatic patients are admitted to the ICU and precautions taken to ensure a secure airway

Serum electrolytes are monitored every 2 h

If seizures are present serum Na^+ concentration can be increased by 4–5 mEq/L in the first hour

Serum Na^+ concentration is increased with either

- Infusion of 3% saline (513 mEq Na/L), which is stopped when serum Na^+ concentration $\geq$120 mEq/L or when symptoms resolve

- Combined loop diuretic and normal saline

- Water restriction alone has no role

In the first 48 h, the serum Na^+ concentration is not increased by greater than 25 mEq/L or corrected to or above normal

In the absence of severe symptoms, serum Na^+ concentration is raised by 0.5 mEq/L/h until 120 mEq/L, and slowly thereafter

Chronic hyponatremia (> 48 h) is not corrected faster than 8 mEq/L in the first 24 h

Liver disease and hypokalemia require a rate of correction closer to 6 mEq/day because of high risk for CPM

(continued)

TABLE 3–26 (Continued)
Caution should be exercised in patients that have reversible defects in renal free water excretion
• Thiazide diuretics that are withdrawn
• Post liver transplant
Abbreviations: ICU, intensive care unit; CPM, central pontine myelinolysis

Table 3–27: Formulas to Calculate Na$^+$ Requirement
Na$^+$ requirement is determined by the following formula: **Na$^+$ requirement**   = (TBW) × (desired serum Na$^+$ concentration   – current serum Na$^+$ concentration)   • TBW is equal to 0.6 times the body weight in men and 0.5 times the body weight in women   • Based on the deficit one then calculates the infusion rate of 3% saline solution
An estimation of the effect of 1 L of any infused solution on the serum [Na$^+$] can be obtained using the following formula: (infusate Na$^+$ concentration – serum Na$^+$ concentration)/   total body water + 1   • Rate of infusate is adjusted to achieve desired increase in serum Na$^+$ concentration
Abbreviations: TBW, total body weight; BW, body weight

TABLE 3–28: Treatment of Hypovolemic Hyponatremia

- Discontinue diuretics, correct GI losses, and expand ECF volume with normal saline

- ECF volume deficit is replaced to eliminate nonosmotic AVP release and promote maximally dilute urine

- Replace one-third of the Na^+ deficit over the first 6–12 h and the remainder over the ensuing 24–48 h
  $$Na^+ \text{ deficit} = \text{(total body water)} \times (140 - \text{current serum } [Na^+])$$

- K^+ deficits must be corrected in the setting of hypokalemia

Abbreviations: GI, gastrointestinal; ECF, extracellular fluid; AVP, arginine vasopressin

TABLE 3–29: Treatment of Euvolemic Hyponatremia

Water restriction is used in the asymptomatic patient

Fluid restriction rarely increases serum $[Na^+]$ by more than 1.5 mEq/L per day

Demeclocycline (600–1200 mg/day) is used for incurable SIADH providing that the patient has normal liver function

Conivaptan hydrochloride injection (20 mg load, followed by 20 mg IV over 24 h) is a V1a/V2 receptor antagonist that was recently approved for SIADH

Oral vasopressin receptor antagonists are in clinical trials and may be useful for therapy of SIADH in the future

Abbreviations: SIADH, syndrome of inappropriate antidiuretic hormone

TABLE 3–30: Treatment of Hypervolemic Hyponatremia

Hypervolemia is managed with salt and water restriction

An increase in cardiac output will suppress AVP release in CHF

Large volume paracentesis, albumin infusion, and water restriction reduces hyponatremia in cirrhotics

Abbreviations: AVP, arginine vasopressin; CHF, congestive heart failure

TABLE 3–31: Example of Change in TBW to Correct Hypervolemic Hyponatremia

A 75-kg man has a total body water of 45 L and a serum $[Na^+]$ of 115 mEq/L

Desired TBW = (actual serum $[Na^+]$/normal serum $[Na^+]$) × current TBW

Desired TBW = (115/140) × 45 L = 36.9 L

45 L – 36.9 L = 8.1 L must be lost to restore serum $[Na^+]$ to 140 mEq/L

Abbreviation: TBW, total body water

TABLE 3–32: Important Concepts in Therapy of Hyponatremia

A fear of CPM delays appropriate correction of severe hyponatremia

- Neurologic sequellae are more commonly related to a slow correction rate rather than rapid correction

- Hypertonic saline should be employed in hyponatremic encephalopathy, even in the absence of seizures

- Prevention of seizures and respiratory arrest are critical to avoid permanent neurologic injury triggered by hypoxia

Rapid correction may occur in patients with the abrupt withdrawal or correction of a stimulus that inhibits free water excretion such as liver transplantation, and elderly women on thiazides in whom the drug is held, and steroid replacement in the patient with panhypopituitarism

- Magnetic resonance imaging best diagnoses CPM (changes are seen 1–2 weeks after onset of signs and symptoms, not immediately)

Patients at high risk for hyponatremic encephalopathy include premenopausal women in the postoperative setting

- Postoperative patients should never receive hypotonic solutions

- Normal saline or Ringers lactate are appropriate

SIADH should never be treated with normal saline alone, as it will result in a further fall in serum Na^+ concentration

- Monitor the patient closely; a falling serum Na^+ concentration with normal saline administration is highly suggestive of SIADH

Abbreviations: CPM, central pontine myelinolysis; SIADH, syndrome of inappropriate antidiuretic hormone

TABLE 3–33: Example of Saline Therapy in SIADH

A patient with SIADH and U_{osm} of 600 mOsm/kg is administered 1 L of normal saline (300 mOsms)

The osmolar load is excreted in 500 mL of urine

300 mOsms/ 600 mOsm/kg (U_{osm}) = 500 mL final urine volume

This results in the generation of 500 mL of free water (rest of the liter) and a fall in serum Na^+ concentration occurs

Abbreviation: U_{osm}, urine osmolality

HYPERNATREMIA

TABLE 3–34: Pathophysiologic Mechanisms of Hypernatremia

Hypernatremia is defined as a serum Na^+ concentration greater than 145 mEq/L

Normally, water loss leads to an increase in osmolality (hypernatremia), which stimulates both AVP and thirst to return osmolality back to normal (see Figure 3–3)

A disturbance in either of these homeostatic mechanisms leads to hypernatremia

Abbreviation: AVP, arginine vasopressin

FIGURE 3–3: Net water loss increases serum osmolality and serum Na$^+$ concentration, thereby stimulating both thirst and AVP production to return water balance to baseline

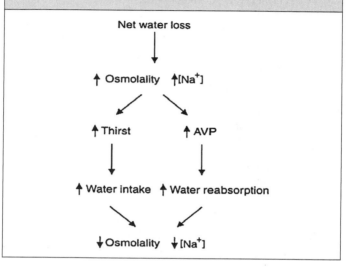

TABLE 3–35: Hypernatremia

Develops in two major settings

- AVP concentration or effect is decreased

- Water intake is less than insensible, GI or renal water losses

  - Inadequate free water intake (access to water or thirst sensation is impaired) in either the presence or absence of a urinary concentrating defect

Hypernatremia can result from salt ingestion or administration of hypertonic saline solutions

The body's major protective mechanisms include thirst and the ability of the kidney to reabsorb water from the urine

Serum osmolality and $[Na^+]$ increase with free water loss

- The rise in serum osmolality has two effects

  - Stimulates thirst

  - Increases AVP release

Normal renal concentration allows for excretion of urine that is four times as concentrated as plasma (1200 mOsm/kg H_2O)

Components of the renal concentrating mechanism include

- Generation of a hypertonic interstitium— Henle's loop acts as a countercurrent multiplier, which dilutes tubular fluid and renders the interstitium hypertonic from cortex to papilla

- AVP secretion—The collecting duct is made permeable to water and allows fluid equilibration with the interstitium

Abbreviations: AVP, arginine vasopressin, GI, gastrointestinal

ETIOLOGY

Hypernatermia due to renal water loss is broadly categorized as either central or nephrogenic diabetes insipidus.

TABLE 3–36: Central DI
• Requires destruction of greater than 80% of vasopressin-producing neurons
• Polyuria (urine volume ranges from 3–15 L/day) is the most common symptom
• Occurs in young patients with nocturia and is associated with a preference for cold water
• Complete central DI is associated with inability to concentrate urine above 200 mOsm/kg with dehydration
• Exogenous AVP increases urine osmolality 100 mOsm/kg above the value achieved following water deprivation
• Partial DI is associated with a smaller concentrating defect
• Increased P_{osm} effectively stimulates thirst, thus serum Na^+ concentration is only slightly elevated
• Central DI is idiopathic or secondary to head trauma, surgery, or neoplasm
■ One-third to one-half are idiopathic with a lymphocytic infiltrate in the posterior pituitary and pituitary stalk (± circulating antibodies against vasopressin-producing neurons)
• Familial central DI is rare and inherited in three ways
■ Autosomal dominant disorder (most common)
■ X-linked recessive inheritance
■ Autosomal recessive disorder (very rare)
Abbreviations: DI, diabetes insipidus; AVP, arginine vasopressin

TABLE 3–37: Nephrogenic DI

Collecting duct does not respond appropriately to AVP

- Inherited forms of nephrogenic DI

- Sex-linked disorder (most common)

  - Caused by mutations in the V2 receptor

- Autosomal dominant and recessive forms

  - Aquaporin-2 gene mutations

  - Results in complete resistance to AVP

- Acquired nephrogenic DI is more common but less severe

  - Chronic kidney disease, hypercalcemia, lithium treatment, obstruction, and hypokalemia are causes

  - Both hypokalemia and hypercalcemia are associated with a significant downregulation of aquaporin-2

  - Drugs may cause a renal concentrating defect

  - Lithium and demeclocycline cause tubular resistance to AVP

  - Amphotericin B and methoxyflurane injure the renal medulla

Abbreviations: DI, diabetes insipidus; AVP, arginine vasopressin

TABLE 3–38: DI Induced by Degradation of AVP by Vasopressinase

Develops in women during the peripartum period

Vasopressinase is produced by the placenta and degrades AVP and oxytocin

It is expressed early in pregnancy and increases in activity throughout gestation

Desmopressin (dD-AVP), which is not degraded by vasopressinase, is effective therapy

After delivery vasopressinase becomes undetectable

Abbreviations: AVP, arginine vasopressin; dD-AVP, 1-deamino-8-D-arginine vasopressin

SIGNS AND SYMPTOMS

Signs and symptoms of hypernatremia are related to cell swelling and shrinking.

TABLE 3–39: Signs and Symptoms of Hypernatremia
Neuromuscular irritability with twitches, hyperreflexia, seizures, coma, and death result from cellular dehydration
The underlying cause of hypernatremia may be the primary symptom early in hypernatremia
• Polyuria and thirst from DI
• Nausea and vomiting or diarrhea with inadequate water access
• Hypodipsia or adipsia (central defect in thirst)
Cellular dehydration in the brain is defended by an increase in brain osmolality
• This is due in part to increases in free amino acids
• The mechanism is unclear, but the phenomenon is referred to as the generation of *idiogenic osmoles*
In children, severe acute hypernatremia (serum Na^+ concentration >160 mEq/L) has a mortality rate of 45%
• Two-thirds of survivors have permanent neurological injury
In adults, acute hypernatremia has a mortality of 75%; chronic hypernatremia has a mortality of 60%
Hypernatremia is often a marker of serious underlying disease
Abbreviation: DI, diabetes insipidus

DIAGNOSIS

TABLE 3–40: Diagnosis of Hypernatremia
Hypernatremia occurs most commonly with hypovolemia, but can occur in association with hypervolemia and euvolemia (see Figure 3–4)
A stepwise approach allows appropriate diagnosis of hypernatremia by assessing thirst, access to water, and the central production of AVP or effect of AVP on the kidney
Step 1 Is thirst intact?
• If the serum Na^+ concentration >147 mEq/L the patient should be thirsty
Step 2 If thirsty, can patient get to water?
• This assesses if the thirst center is intact and if the patient has access to water or other hypotonic solutions
Step 3 Evaluate the hypothalamic-pituitary-renal axis
• This involves an examination of urine osmolality
Abbreviation: AVP, arginine vasopressin

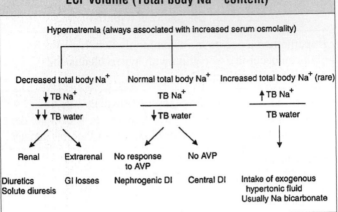

FIGURE 3–4: Hypernatremia is classified initially based on ECF volume (Total body Na$^+$ content)

Hypernatremia (always associated with increased serum osmolality)

Decreased total body Na$^+$	Normal total body Na$^+$	Increased total body Na$^+$ (rare)
↓ TB Na$^+$	TB Na$^+$	↑ TB Na$^+$
↓↓ TB water	↓ TB water	TB water

Renal   Extrarenal   No response to AVP   No AVP

Diuretics   GI losses   Nephrogenic DI   Central DI   Intake of exogenous
Solute diuresis   hypertonic fluid
                                                   Usually Na bicarbonate

TABLE 3–41: Hypothalamic-Pituitary Axis

An intact axis maximally stimulates AVP release and results in U_{osm} > 700 mOsm/kg when serum Na^+ concentration >147 mEq/L

Free water losses are often extrarenal if urine osmolality >700 mOsm/kg

U_{osm} less than plasma indicates that there is renal source of free water loss (central or nephrogenic DI)

Differentiate by the response to exogenous AVP [subcutaneous aqueous vasopressin (5 units) or intranasal dD-AVP (10 mcg)]

- Increases urine osmolality by ≥50% in central DI

- No effect on urine osmolality in nephrogenic DI

U_{osm} in the intermediate range (300–600 mOsm/kg) may be secondary to psychogenic polydipsia, osmotic diuresis, and partial central or nephrogenic DI

Psychogenic polydipsia is associated with a mildly decreased rather than increased serum Na^+ concentration

Partial central and nephrogenic DI may require a water deprivation test to distinguish

Abbreviations: AVP, arginine vasopressin; U_{osm}, urine osmolality; DI, diabetes insipidus; dD-AVP, 1-deamino-8-D-arginine vasopressin

TABLE 3–42: Water Deprivation Test

Water is prohibited, urine volume and osmolality is measured hourly, and serum Na^+ concentration and osmolality is measured every 2h

The test is stopped if any of the following occur

- U_{osm} reaches normal levels

- P_{osm} reaches 300 mOsm/kg

- U_{osm} is stable on two successive readings despite a rising serum osmolality

- In the last two circumstances exogenous AVP is administered and the U_{osm} and volume measured

  - Partial central DI has urine osmolality increase >50 mOsm/kg

  - Partial nephrogenic DI has no or minimal increase in urine osmolality

Abbreviations: U_{osm}, urine osmolality; P_{osm}, plasma osmolality; AVP, arginine vasopressin; DI, diabetes insipidus

TREATMENT

Table 3–43: General Treatment of Hypernatremia

Treatment of hypernatremia is divided into two parts

- Restore plasma tonicity to normal and correct Na^+ imbalances by correcting the water deficit

- Provide treatment directed at the underlying disorder

Table 3–44: Therapy of Hypernatremia: Correcting the Water Deficit

Water deficits are restored slowly to avoid sudden shifts in brain cell volume

- Increased oral water intake

- Intravenous administration of hypotonic solution

Serum Na^+ concentration should not be lowered faster than 8–10 mEq/day

The formula below calculates the initial amount of free water replacement needed (not ongoing losses)

Ongoing renal free water losses should be added to the replacement calculation

Renal free water losses are calculated as the electrolyte-free water clearance, dividing urine into two components

- Isotonic component (the volume needed to excrete Na^+ and K^+ at their concentration in serum)

- Electrolyte-free water

Formula for electrolyte-free water clearance

- **Urine volume** = $C_{Electrolytes} + C_{H_2O}$

- $C_{Electrolytes}$ = (Urine $[Na^+] + [K^+]$)/serum $[Na^+]$) × urine volume

- C_{H_2O} = the volume of urine from which the electrolytes were removed during elaboration of a hypotonic urine

TABLE 3–45: Example of Treatment of Hypernatremia

A 70-kg male with a history of central DI is found unconscious; serum $[Na^+]$ = 160 mEq/L and urine output is 500 mL/h

Urine electrolytes reveal the following values: $[Na^+]$ = 60 mEq/L, $[K^+]$ = 20 mEq/L and U_{osm} = 180 mOsm/kg

How much water is required to correct the serum $[Na^+]$ to 140 mEq/L?

$$\text{Water needed (L)} = (0.6 \text{ body weight in kg}) \ ((\text{actual } [Na^+]/\text{desired } [Na^+]) - 1)$$
$$= (0.6 \times 70)((160/140) - 1)$$
$$= 42 \times 0.14 \text{ or } 6L$$

If serum $[Na^+]$ were decreased by 8 mEq/L in the first 24 h, then 2.4 L of water (100 mL/h) would be required for the deficit

The serum $[Na^+]$ increases with this solution because the calculation did not include the large ongoing free water loss in urine

To include renal free water losses one must calculate the electrolyte-free water clearance as illustrated

$$C_{\textbf{Electrolytes}} = ((\text{Urine } [Na^+] + [K^+])/\text{serum } [Na^+]) \times \text{urine volume}$$
$$C_{\textbf{H}_2\textbf{O}} = \text{Urine volume} - C_{\text{Electrolytes}}$$

Ongoing renal free water losses of 250 mL/h are added to the replacement solution (100 mL/h), giving a total of 350 mL/h required to correct the serum Na^+ concentration

Abbreviation: DI, diabetes insipidus

TABLE 3–46: Therapy of Hypernatremia: Based on the Underlying Disorder

Nephrogenic diabetes insipidus

- Reduce urine volume and renal free water excretion

- Urine volume can be reduced by

  - Decreasing osmolar intake (protein or salt restriction)

  - Increasing U_{osm}

- **Urine volume** = solute intake or excretion (the same in the steady state)/ U_{osm}

- Thiazide diuretics inhibit urinary dilution and increase urine osmolality

- Nonsteroidal anti-inflammatory drugs (NSAIDs) inhibit synthesis of renal prostaglandins (which normally antagonize AVP effect) and increase concentrating ability

Electrolyte disturbances

- Both hypokalemia and hypercalcemia reduce urinary concentration and should be corrected

Lithium-induced nephrogenic diabetes insipidus

- Stop lithium and/or use amiloride to ameliorate DI by preventing entry of lithium into the CCD

Central diabetes insipidus

- Intranasal dD-AVP (5 μg at bedtime) is initiated and titrated up (5–20 μg once or twice daily)

- Oral desmopressin is an alternative (0.1 mg tablet = 2.5–5.0 μg of nasal spray)

- Drugs that increase AVP release (clofibrate) or enhance its effect (chlorpropamide, carbamazepine) can be added

Abbreviations: U_{osm}, urine osmolality; NSAIDs, nonsteroidal anti-inflammatory drugs; AVP, arginine vasopressin; DI, diabetes insipidus; CCD, cortical collecting duct, dD-AVP, 1-deamino-8-D-arginine vasopressin

TABLE 3–47: Treatment of Central DI		
Condition	**Drug**	**Dose**
Complete DI		
	dD-AVP	5–20 µg intranasal q 12–24 h 0.1–0.4 mg orally q12–24 h
Incomplete DI		
	Chlorpropamide	125–500 mg/day
	Carbamazepine	100–300 mg BID
	Clofibrate	500 mg QID
Abbreviations: DI, diabetes insipidus; BID, twice a day; QID, four times a day; dD-AVP, 1-deamino-8-D-arginine vasopressin		

4
Diuretics

INTRODUCTION

TABLE 4–1: Basics of Diuretics

Kidneys regulate ECF volume by modulating NaCl and water excretion

Diuretics increase the amount of urine formed, due primarily to inhibition of Na^+ and water reabsorption along the nephron

Diuretics are used to treat a variety of clinical disease states:

- Hypertension, edema, congestive heart failure, hyperkalemia, and hypercalcemia

Abbreviation: ECF, extracellular fluid volume

TABLE 4–2: Renal Regulation of NaCl and Water Excretion

Na^+ absorption is regulated by several factors:

- Hormones (renin, AII, aldosterone, atrial natriuretic peptide, prostaglandins, and endothelin)

- Physical properties (mean arterial pressure, peritubular capillary pressure, and renal interstitial pressure) affect handling of Na^+ and water

Na^+ reabsorption is driven by Na^+-K^+ ATPase located on basolateral membrane

- It provides energy for transporters located on the apical membrane that reabsorb Na^+ from glomerular filtrate

Cell-specific transporters are present on these tubular cells

- Diuretics enhance renal Na^+ and water excretion by inhibiting these transporters at different nephron sites (see Figure 4–1)

Abbreviation: AII, angiotensin II

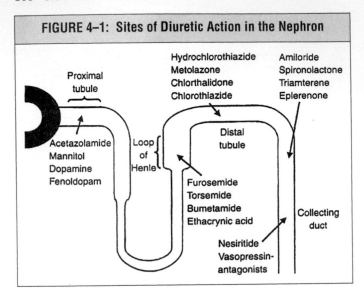

FIGURE 4–1: Sites of Diuretic Action in the Nephron

TABLE 4–3: General Characteristics of Diuretics

Act on the luminal surface (except spironolactone or eplerenone) and must enter tubular fluid to be effective

Secretion across the proximal tubule via organic acid or base transporters is the primary mode of entry (except mannitol, which undergoes glomerular filtration)

Potency depends on the following:

- Drug delivery to the nephron site of action

- Glomerular filtration rate

- State of the effective arterial blood volume (congestive heart failure, cirrhosis, and nephrosis)

- Treatment with medications such as NSAIDs and probenecid (reduce potency)

Diuretics have adverse effects, some that are common to all diuretics and others that are unique

Abbreviation: NSAIDs, nonsteroidal anti-inflammatory drugs

SITES OF DIURETIC ACTION IN KIDNEY

TABLE 4–4: Proximal Tubule
Na$^+$ delivered via glomerular filtration
Na$^+$ transport in the proximal tubular cell is driven by Na$^+$-K$^+$ ATPase activity
• Energy derived from ATP moves three Na$^+$ ions out of the cell in exchange for two K$^+$ ions
• A reduction of intracellular Na$^+$ concentration results
• Na$^+$ moves down its electrochemical gradient from tubular lumen into the cell via the Na$^+$-H$^+$ exchanger in exchange for H$^+$ that moves out
• H$^+$ secretion is associated with reclamation of filtered bicarbonate
Abbreviation: ATP, adenosine triphosphate

TABLE 4–5: Proximal Tubule Diuretics
Mannitol
Employed for prophylaxis to prevent ischemic or nephrotoxic renal injury and to reduce cerebral edema
Nonmetabolizable osmotic agent that is freely filtered, raises intratubular osmolality and drags water and Na^+ into the tubule
Active only when given intravenously
Acts within 10 min and has a $t_{1/2}$ of approximately 1.2 h in patients with normal renal function
Toxicity develops when filtration of mannitol is impaired, as in renal dysfunction
• Retained mannitol increases P_{osm}
▪ Exacerbates CHF, induces hyponatremia, and causes a hyperoncotic syndrome
▪ Contraindicated in patients with CHF and moderate to severe kidney disease
Nausea and vomiting, and headache are adverse effects
Acetazolamide (primarily proximal tubular)
A CA inhibitor that alkalinizes the urine, prevents and treats altitude sickness, and decreases intraocular pressure in glaucoma
Disrupts bicarbonate reabsorption by impairing the conversion of carbonic acid (H_2CO_3) into CO_2 and H_2O in tubular fluid and within renal tubular epithelial cells
• Excess bicarbonate in the tubular lumen associates with Na^+ and exits the proximal tubule

(continued)

TABLE 4–5 (Continued)
Exerts its effect within 1/2 h and maintains a $t_{1/2}$ of 13 h
Over time the effect of these drugs diminishes due to the reduction in plasma and filtered bicarbonate
Metabolic consequences include nonanion gap metabolic acidosis and hypokalemia
• Should be avoided in cirrhotics (increases serum NH_3) or with hypokalemia
Other adverse effects include drowsiness, fatigue, lethargy, paresthesias, and bone marrow suppression
Proximal tubule diuretics are weak diuretics because downstream nephron segments reabsorb Na^+
Abbreviations: P_{osm}, plasma osmolality; CHF, congestive heart failure; CA, carbonic anhydrase

TABLE 4–6: Thick Ascending Limb of the Loop of Henle
In this segment, the Na^+-K^+-$2Cl^-$ cotransporter on the apical membrane, powered by Na^+-K^+ ATPase on the basolateral membrane reabsorbs the following:
• Significant NaCl (20–30% of the filtered Na^+ load)
• K^+, Ca^{2+}, and Mg^{2+}

TABLE 4–7: Loop of Henle Diuretics

Loop diuretics include furosemide, bumetanide, torsemide, and ethacrynic acid (most potent diuretics)

These drugs are used primarily to treat

- Congestive heart failure

- Cirrhosis-associated ascites and edema

- Nephrotic syndrome

- Hypercalcemia (with normal saline)

- Hypertension (moderate to severe kidney disease)

- Hyponatremia in setting of SIADH

Loop diuretics are given via either the oral or IV route

- Act within 20–30 min and have a $t_{1/2}$ of approximately 1–1.5 h (torsemide; $t_{1/2}$ of 3–4 h)

- In healthy subjects, there is no difference in urine volume, natriuresis or K^+ and Cl^- excretion

- Peak natriuretic action with oral administration is 75 min; while IV administration is 30 min

In CKD, dose of loop diuretic to promote effective natriuresis is higher than with normal kidney function

- Lower GFR reduces filtered Na^+ load (filtered Na^+ with GFR of 100 mL/min is 15 mEq/min, whereas it is 0.15 mEq/min with GFR of 10 mL/min)

- In advanced CKD, maximal diuretic response to IV furosemide occurs at 160–200 mg

- Decreased delivery of loop diuretic to its site of action limits efficacy at lower administered doses with CKD

(continued)

TABLE 4–7 (Continued)

In normal subjects, the dose equivalency for loop diuretics is
Bumetanide 1 *mg* = Torsemide 10 *mg* = Furosemide 40 *mg*

Abbreviations: SIADH, syndrome of inappropriate antidiuretic
hormone; IV, intravenous; CKD, chronic kidney disease; GFR,
glomerular filtration rate

TABLE 4–8: Ceiling Doses of IV and Oral Loop Diuretics in Various Clinical Conditions

The maximum dose of each drug varies based on the indication
and the underlying disease state

Ceiling dose is defined as the dose that provides maximal
inhibition of NaCl reabsorption (plateau in the diuretic
dose-response curve)

Clinical Condition	Furosemide (mg)		Bumetanide (mg)		Torsemide (mg)	
	IV	PO	IV	PO	IV	PO
Kidney disease						
GFR 20–50 mL/min	80	60–80	2–3	2–3	20–50	20–50
GFR <20 mL/min	200	240	8–10	8–10	50–100	50–100
CHF	40–80	160–240	2–3	2–3	20–50	20–50
Nephrosis	120		3		50	50
Cirrhosis	40–80	80–160	1	1–2	10–20	20–50

Abbreviations: IV, intravenous; PO, oral; GFR, glomerular
filtration rate; CHF, congestive heart failure

TABLE 4–9: Adverse Effects of Loop Diuretics

Hypokalemia, hypocalcemia, hypomagnesemia, volume contraction (shock), and metabolic alkalosis

Precipitate hepatorenal syndrome in cirrhotics and lethal arrhythmias from hypokalemia in patients on digoxin

Ethacrynic acid is associated with severe ototoxicity

Furosemide, torsemide, and bumetanide are contraindicated in patients with sulfonamide allergy

Mild hyperglycemia occurs due to inhibition of insulin release

Blood dyscrasia (thrombocytopenia, agranulocytosis)

TABLE 4–10: Distal Convoluted Tubule

DCT reabsorbs 5–10% of the filtered Na^+ load

DCT contains the thiazide-sensitive Na-Cl cotransporter (NCC), which reabsorbs Na^+ and Cl^-

Abbreviations: DCT, distal convoluted tubule; NCC, Na-Cl cotransporter

TABLE 4–11: DCT Diuretics
Thiazide and thiazide-like diuretics inhibit NCC in DCT
Used primarily to treat:
• Hypertension
• Osteoporosis and nephrolithiasis
Thiazides are used in combination with loop diuretics to enhance natriuresis in patients that develop diuretic resistance
Available as both oral (HCTZ and metolazone) and IV preparations (chlorothiazide)
They are well absorbed following oral administration with an onset of action within 1 h
The $t_{1/2}$ is variable between drugs with duration of action from 6–48 h
• HCTZ dose ranges from 12.5–50 mg/day
• Metolazone dosing (2.5 mg/day to 10 mg twice daily)
Bioavailability is reduced with CKD, liver disease, and CHF
• GFR < 25–40 mL/min limits drug delivery to DCT
• Metolazone maintains efficacy at lower GFRs
Abbreviations: DCT, distal convoluted tubule; NCC, Na-Cl cotransporter; HCTZ, hydrochlorothiazide; IV, intravenous; CKD, chronic kidney disease; CHF, congestive heart failure; GFR, glomerular filtration rate

TABLE 4–12: Adverse Effects of DCT Diuretics

Hypokalemia, hypomagnesemia, hyponatremia, and metabolic alkalosis

Patients with cirrhosis are at risk for encephalopathy from hypokalemia and elevated plasma NH_3 concentrations

Hypercalcemia develops in patients with $1°$ hyperparathyroidism and those that are bed bound

Hypersensitivity reactions include pancreatitis, hemolytic anemia, and thrombocytopenia

Increased proximal uric acid reabsorption promotes hyperuricemia and gout

Abbreviation: DCT, distal convoluted tubule

TABLE 4–13: Cortical Collecting Duct

CCD reabsorbs 1–3% of the filtered Na^+ load

Reabsorption of NaCl and K^+ secretion in the principal cell is controlled primarily by aldosterone and plasma K^+ concentration

Na^+ is reabsorbed through a sodium channel (ENaC) and K^+ secreted through a potassium channel (ROMK)

All drugs that act in the CCD are weak diuretics

Abbreviations: CCD, cortical collecting duct; ENaC, epithelial Na^+ channel; ROMK, rat outer medullary potassium

TABLE 4–14: CCD Diuretics

Mineralocorticoid receptor blockers (spironolactone and eplerenone) blunt aldosterone-induced NaCl reabsorption and K^+ secretion

They treat hypertension in both 1° and 2° aldosteronism

Reduce edema and ascites in patients with cirrhosis

Improve cardiac dysfunction in patients with CHF (EF < 40%)

Spironolactone has excellent oral bioavailability

- Undergoes hepatic metabolism ($t_{1/2}$ of 20 h) and requires 2 days to become effective

- The dose range is 25–200 mg/day

Eplerenone has excellent oral bioavailability

- It has a shorter $t_{1/2}$ (4–6), is metabolized by the liver (CYP3A4), and is excreted (67%) by the kidney

- Dose range is 25–100 mg/day, with twice/day dosing most effective

ENaC blockers (amiloride and triamterene) reduce NaCl reabsorption and K^+ secretion

Reduce K^+ losses associated with other diuretics and prevent hypokalemia

Are given in combination with thiazide diuretics (HCTZ and amiloride, HCTZ and triamterene)

Amiloride is well absorbed with oral administration ($t_{1/2}$ of 6 h and is excreted renally)

Triamterene is well absorbed and has a short $t_{1/2}$ (3 h)

Abbreviations: CCD, cortical collecting duct; CHF, congestive heart failure; ENaC, epithelial Na^+ channel; HCTZ, hydrochlorothiazide

TABLE 4–15: Adverse Effects of CCD Diuretics

Hyperkalemia and hyperchloremic metabolic acidosis

- Moderate to severe kidney disease increases risk

- K^+ supplements or medications that impair K^+ homeostasis such as ACE inhibitors, ARBs, and NSAIDs enhance risk

- Patients with diabetes mellitus (hyporeninemic hypoaldosteronism) and tubulointerstitial kidney disease are at increased risk

Spironolactone causes gynecomastia, hirsutism, menstrual irregularities, and testicular atrophy (androgen receptor binding), these occur less often with eplerenone (specific for mineralocorticoid receptor)

Amiloride and triamterene can cause nausea and vomiting, rarely a metabolic acidosis and hyponatremia may occur

Amiloride promotes glucose intolerance, while triamterene causes megaloblastic anemia and urinary crystal formation/nephrolithiasis

Abbreviations: CCD, cortical collecting duct; ACE, angiotensin converting enzyme; ARB, angiotensin receptor blocker; NSAID, nonsteroidal anti-inflammatory drug

DIURETIC RESISTANCE

TABLE 4–16: Approach to the Patient with Diuretic Resistance
Step 1 Define diuretic resistance as failure to resolve edema or hypertension with standard diuretic doses
Step 2 Identify cause and type of edema   • Differentiate generalized renal-related edema from localized edema due to venous or lymphatic obstruction   • Cyclic edema (occurs only in women) and interstitial edema due to fluid redistributed from plasma compartment (Ca^{2+} channel blockers) is not amenable to diuretic therapy
Step 3 Examine for incomplete therapy of the primary disorder   • Clinical disorders associated with impaired diuretic response include CHF, cirrhosis with ascites, nephrotic syndrome, hypertension, and kidney disease   • In patients with severe congestive cardiomyopathies and decompensated CHF, an IV inotropic agent (dobutamine) improves cardiac pump function and renal perfusion   • Excessive reductions in arterial BP may induce diuretic resistance; allowing the BP to increase can be beneficial
Step 4 Assess patient compliance with salt restricted diet and diuretic regimen   • Diet (ingestion of canned foods or fast foods) history is often illuminating   • Patients drink large amounts of certain beverages (gatorade), which can overcome diuretic effect   • Adverse effects from diuretics, such as impotence and muscle cramps, may promote noncompliance

TABLE 4–16 (Continued)

Step 5 Consider pharmacokinetic alterations of the diuretic
- Ineffective diuresis results from poor drug absorption as seen with edematous (bowel edema) or poor cardiac output states, vascular disease of the intestinal tree, and cirrhosis (inadequate blood flow for drug absorption)
- Reduced GFR decreases the concentration of diuretic that reaches the site of action in the tubular lumen

Step 6 Consider pharmacodynamic alterations of the diuretic regimen, due to renal Na^+ retention from various mechanisms
- Activation of the RAAS and SNS reduces diuretic response by lowering GFR and increasing NaCl reabsorption along nephron segments
- Stimulation of the RAAS and SNS occurs for two reasons
  - Cirrhosis, CHF, and nephrotic syndrome decrease effective arterial blood volume, activating the RAAS and SNS that enhance Na^+ reabsorption
  - Diuretics reflexively activate the RAAS and SNS, perpetuating diuretic resistance
- Compensatory changes in distal nephron cells following chronic therapy with loop diuretics induce resistance
  - Increased delivery of NaCl to the DCT induces hypertrophy/hyperplasia of tubular cells and increases density of both Na^+-K^+ ATPase pumps and NCC cotransporters, enhancing the intrinsic capacity of the DCT to reabsorb Na^+ and Cl^-

Step 7 Explore for adverse drug interactions that blunt diuresis
- NSAIDs impair intrarenal synthesis of prostaglandins, which maintain GFR and block NaCl reabsorption in all nephron segments

(continued)

TABLE 4–16 (Continued)
• Diuretic resistance from NSAIDs develops in certain patients (hypertension, CHF, cirrhosis, nephrotic syndrome, CKD) from impaired natriuresis • Probenecid, cimetidine, and trimethoprim compete with diuretics for PCT transport pathways, reducing diuretic delivery to their sites of action
Abbreviations: CHF, congestive heart failure; IV, intravenous; GFR, glomerular filtration rate; RAAS, renin-angiotensin-aldosterone system; SNS, sympathetic nervous system; DCT, distal convoluted tubule; NSAID, nonsteroidal anti-inflammatory drug; CKD, chronic kidney disease; PCT, proximal convoluted tubule

CLINICAL CONDITIONS ASSOCIATED WITH DIURETIC RESISTANCE

TABLE 4–17: Congestive Heart Failure and Na^+ Retention
The hemodynamics of CHF promote Na^+ and water retention from reduced renal perfusion, activated RAAS and SNS, and enhanced AVP release
The severity of cardiac dysfunction dictates the degree of tubular NaCl and fluid reabsorption
Treatment is directed at improving cardiac function and assessing for other factors causing diuretic resistance
Impaired GI absorption contributes to suboptimal response in CHF
• Bowel edema, reduced bowel wall perfusion, and disturbed GI motility reduces absorption
Abbreviations: CHF, congestive heart failure; RAAS, renin-angiotensin-aldosterone system; SNS, sympathetic nervous system; AVP, arginine vasopressin; GI, gastrointestinal

TABLE 4–18: Diuretic Resistance Associated with Nephrotic Syndrome

Na^+ and fluid retention in patients with nephrotic syndrome develops from the following:

- Activated RAAS and SNS, increased concentrations of AVP, and direct stimulation of NHE3 transport in PCT by excessive urinary protein concentration

- Renal dysfunction reduces the filtered load of NaCl while primary renal Na^+ retention also causes edema formation

Hypoalbuminemia increases the volume of distribution of diuretics, reducing the concentration of drug in the circulation and the amount delivered to the kidney

Hypoalbuminemia reduces drug transport into urine independent of renal delivery (loss of albumin stimulation of organic anion transport pathway)

Collecting duct resistance to atrial natriuretic peptide stimulated natriuresis

Excessive albumin concentrations in tubule fluid bind diuretics and reduce free urinary drug levels

Abbreviations: RAAS, renin-angiotensin-aldosterone system; SNS, sympathetic nervous system; AVP, arginine vasopressin; PCT, proximal convoluted tubule

TABLE 4–19: Edema Formation in Cirrhosis

Edema formation and ascites occur with advanced cirrhosis or during acute decompensation of chronic liver disease

Enhanced proximal tubular Na^+ and fluid reabsorption, stimulated by activated RAAS and SNS, reduces Na^+ delivery to more distal sites where loop diuretics act

Secondary aldosteronism stimulates avid NaCl uptake by DCT and CCD

Intestinal edema limits drug absorption, while hypoalbuminemia increases volume of distribution

Reductions in GFR also contribute to suboptimal diuresis

Spontaneous bacterial peritonitis and low BP exacerbate cirrhotic hemodynamics and enhance diuretic resistance

Abbreviations: RAAS, renin-angiotensin-aldosterone system; SNS, sympathetic nervous system; DCT, distal convoluted tubule; CCD, cortical collecting duct; GFR, glomerular filtration rate; BP, blood pressure

TABLE 4–20: Na^+ Contribution to Hypertension

Essential hypertension is a disturbance in renal salt handling. Salt restriction and diuretics are the initial management options.

Dietary salt excess (processed, canned, or fast foods) causes diuretic resistance in one-third of patients

RAAS activation prior to diuretic therapy is worsened by further diuretic treatment, promoting renal NaCl retention and peripheral vasoconstriction

Abbreviation: RAAS, renin-angiotensin-aldosterone system

TABLE 4–21: Diminished Diuretic Effect in Kidney Disease
As GFR declines, diuretic effects diminish; escalating doses of diuretics are required to promote an adequate diuresis
Reduced filtered Na^+ and decreased drug delivery to site of action are primarily responsible for diuretic resistance
Endogenous organic anions (accumulate in uremia) compete with diuretics for organic anion transporters
• Secretion of drug into tubular fluid is reduced and the diuretic can't reach its site of action
Abbreviation: GFR, glomerular filtration rate

TREATMENT OF DIURETIC RESISTANCE

TABLE 4–22: Oral versus IV Diuretic Therapy
Patients responding marginally to oral loop diuretics benefit from dose adjustment or switch to IV therapy
Initial treatment of patients with diuretic resistance is escalation of the oral dose of loop diuretic
Dosing interval for loop diuretics must be no longer than 8–12 h (based on time of drug effect), or a rebound increase in Na^+ reabsorption (post-diuretic NaCl retention) will occur
IV therapy is often required to restore diuretic efficacy in patients with absorptive problems such as bowel edema, altered GI motility, and reduced bowel perfusion
Drug-related toxicity limits high-dose loop diuretic therapy
• Ototoxicity is typically reversible; sometimes permanent
• Myalgias complicate high dose bumetanide therapy
Abbreviations: IV, intravenous; GI, gastrointestinal

TABLE 4–23: Advantages of Continuous Diuretic Infusions
Patients responding marginally to high dose IV loop diuretics benefit from continuous diuretic infusion
Trough concentrations of loop diuretic are avoided and post-diuretic NaCl retention is averted
Continuous infusions achieve 30% more natriuresis for the same IV bolus dose
Efficacy is greatest for bumetanide (shortest $t_{1/2}$) and least for torsemide (longest $t_{1/2}$)
Dose titration is more easily achieved
Toxicity is reduced with continuous infusion as high peak concentrations of bolus therapy are avoided
Abbreviation: IV, intravenous

TABLE 4–24: Dosing Guidelines for Continuous Infusions of Loop Diuretics		
Diuretic	**Bolus Dose (mg)**	**Infusion Rate (mg/kg/hour)**
Furosemide	20–80	2–100 (up to 1.0)
Torsemide	25	1–50 (up to 0.5)
Bumetanide	1.0	0.2–2 (up to 0.02)

TABLE 4–25: Synergistic Effect of Combined Loop and DCT Diuretic

Addition of a second diuretic class overcomes diuretic resistance

The patient failing the ceiling dose of loop diuretic benefits from the addition of a thiazide diuretic

- The longer half-life of a thiazide diuretic attenuates the post-diuretic NaCl retention of a loop diuretic

- High dose IV chlorothiazide improves Na^+ delivery from the PCT to the TALH by inhibiting carbonic anhydrase

- Thiazides improve loop diuretic efficacy by blunting NaCl reabsorption by hypertrophic and hyperplastic DCT cells

- Patients with CHF, cirrhosis, and nephrotic syndrome benefit from a CCD diuretic (spironolactone, eplerenone), which modulates the activated RAAS

- PCT or CCD diuretics can be added to loop diuretics depending on the underlying clinical condition, like acetazolamide for metabolic alkalosis

Abbreviations: IV, intravenous; PCT, proximal convoluted tubule; TALH, thick ascending limb of Henle; DCT, distal convoluted tubule; CHF, congestive heart failure; CCD, cortical collecting duct; RAAS, renin-angiotensin-aldosterone system

TABLE 4–26: Dosing Guidelines for Diuretics Added to Loop Diuretics	
Class of Diuretic	**Dose Range (mg/day)**
Proximal tubule diuretics	
Acetazolamide	250–375; up to 500 (IV)
Distal convoluted tubule diuretic	
Chlorothiazide	500–1000 (IV)
Metolazone	2.5–10 (PO)
Hydrochlorothiazide	25–100 (PO)
Collecting tubule diuretics	
Amiloride	5–10 (PO)
Spironolactone	100–200 (PO)
Eplerenone	25–100 (PO)
Abbreviation: IV, intravenous; PO, oral	

TABLE 4–27: Monitoring Combination Diuretic Therapy

Combination diuretic therapy can promote vigorous diuresis with severe hypovolemia, as well as electrolyte disturbances

Cautious prescription and monitoring for side effects is needed

Patients should perform daily weights and contact their physician with any changes greater than 2 lb/day

Electrolytes and renal function should be measured within 5–7 days of initiating combination therapy

When adding a thiazide diuretic to a loop diuretic it is wise to give the thiazide for only the first 2–3 days of the week, rather than as an open ended daily prescription to limit overdiuresis

Several cardiovascular drugs increase renal blood flow, GFR, and natriuresis through both cardiovascular and direct renal effects.

TABLE 4–28: Cardiovascular Drugs Employed to Enhance Diuresis
Dopamine infusion
• A dose of 1–3 µg/kg/min stimulates renal dopamine receptors (DA_1 and DA_2) and enhances natriuresis
• A dose of 5 mcg/kg/min stimulates beta-adrenergic receptors and increases cardiac output enhancing diuresis
• Doses greater than 5 µg/kg/min cause tachycardia and increase systemic vascular resistance
• Natriuresis wanes after 24 h of dopamine infusion
• Addition of dopamine to diuretics is of limited benefit and is associated with potentially serious tachyarrhythmias
Fenoldopam infusion
• A selective DA_1 receptor agonist
• Approved to treat urgent or malignant hypertension
• Lowers blood pressure through systemic vasodilation
• Induces natriuresis by binding renal DA_1 receptors (inhibiting NHE3)
• Renal effects are 6 times more potent than dopamine

TABLE 4–28 (Continued)

Dobutamine

- An inotrope that does not cause systemic or mesenteric vasoconstriction

- Increases cardiac output and reflexively reduces systemic vascular resistance

- Improves renal blood flow in the patient with congestive cardiomyopathy and enhances urinary Na^+ excretion

- Dopamine and dobutamine produce synergistic effects

Atrial and brain natriuretic peptide

- Both peptides are released in response to the high filling pressures associated with heart failure

- These peptides are natriuretic and diuretic and lower BP by reducing RAAS, SNS, and endothelin activity

- Used to treat CHF resistant to other medical management

- Diuresis and natriuresis occurs through multiple effects

  - Increases in GFR (increased Na^+ filtration)

  - Stimulation of cyclic GMP in inner medullary collecting duct, closing nonspecific cation channels

  - Stimulation of dopamine secretion in PCT

  - Inhibition of AII and aldosterone production

(continued)

TABLE 4–28 (Continued)
• Nesiritide (BNP) is administered as follows:
▪ IV bolus (2 mcg/kg) is given initially
▪ Continuous infusion (0.01 mcg/kg/min) is titrated to a maximum dose of 0.03 mcg/kg/min
▪ This therapy increases natriuresis and cardiac index, lowers cardiac filling pressure and reduces blood pressure
▪ Reversible hypotension limits therapy
Vasopressin (V_2) receptor antagonists
• Target the renal AVP receptor
• V_2 antagonists facilitate a water diuresis
• IV conivaptan hydrochloride (V_{1A}/V_2 antagonist) was recently approved for therapy of SIADH
• Enhance free water clearance and treat various forms of hyponatremia, including that caused by diuretics
Abbreviations: RAAS, renin-angiotensin-aldosterone system; SNS, sympathetic nervous system; CHF, congestive heart failure; GFR, glomerular filtration rate; GMP, guanosine monophosphate; PCT, proximal convoluted tubule; BNP, brain natriuretic peptide; IV, intravenous; AVP, arginine vasopressin; TALH, thick ascending limb of Henle; SIADH, syndrome of inappropriate antidiuretic hormone

5
Disorders of K$^+$ Balance
(Hypo- and Hyperkalemia)

INTRODUCTION

TABLE 5–1: Cellular Effects of High Intracellular K$^+$ Concentration
Disorders of K$^+$ balance are associated with significant morbidity and mortality due to effects on a number of cellular functions
A high cellular concentration is required to maintain normal function of a number of cellular processes
• Nucleic acid and protein synthesis
• Regulation of cell volume, pH, cell growth, and enzyme activation
A high intracellular [K$^+$] is necessary for the maintenance of the resting membrane potential (E_m)
• The E_m in concert with the threshold membrane potential sets the stage for action potential generation
• Action potential generation is required for proper functioning of excitable tissues

TABLE 5–2: Basics of K$^+$ Homeostasis

K$^+$ is the predominant intracellular cation in the body

Regulation of K$^+$ homeostasis is achieved through cellular K$^+$ shifts and renal K$^+$ excretion

- Disturbances in these homeostatic mechanisms result in either hypokalemia or hyperkalemia

Hypo- and hyperkalemia disrupt action potential formation and promote various clinical symptoms and physical findings based on the following:

- Neuromuscular dysfunction

- Inhibition of normal cell enzymatics

Rapid recognition and treatment of these K$^+$ disorders is required to avoid serious morbidity and mortality

K+ HOMEOSTASIS

TABLE 5–3: Total Body K+ Stores
K+ homeostasis involves maintenance of total body K+ stores within the normal range
Total body K+ stores in an adult are between 3000 and 4000 mEq
• 50–60 mEq/kg body weight
Total body K+ content is also influenced by age and sex
• Compared with the young, the elderly have 20% less total body K+ content
• Females have 25% less total body K+ than males
K+ is readily absorbed from the GI tract and subsequently distributed in cells of muscle, liver, bone, and red blood cells
Maintenance of total body K+ stores within narrow limits is achieved by:
• Regulation of K+ distribution between ECF and ICF
• Zero net balance between input and output
K+ is an intracellular cation (98% of body K+ located in ICF)
• Intracellular K+ concentration (145 mEq/L)
• Extracellular K+ concentration (4–5 mEq/L)
Dietary K+ is excreted mainly in urine (90%) and in feces (10%)

TABLE 5–3 (Continued)
The serum K^+ concentration is an index of K^+ balance
• It reasonably reflects total body K^+ content
• In disease states, serum $[K^+]$ may not always reflect total body K^+ stores
Abbreviations: GI, gastrointestinal; ECF, extracellular fluid; ICF, intracellular fluid

ROLE OF K⁺ IN THE RESTING MEMBRANE POTENTIAL

TABLE 5–4: Role of K^+ in Resting Membrane Potential (E_m)
The location of K^+ and Na^+ in their respective compartments is maintained by Na^+-K^+ ATPase action in the cell membrane
The Na^+-K^+ ATPase hydrolyzes ATP to create the energy required to pump Na^+ out and K^+ into the cell in 3:2 ratio
K^+ moves out of cells at a rate dependent on the electrochemical gradient, creating the E_m
The *Goldman-Hodgkin-Katz equation* calculates the membrane potential on the inside of the membrane using Na^+ and K^+

TABLE 5–5: Three Factors Determine Resting Membrane Potential (E$_m$)

Electrical charge of each ion
Membrane permeability to each ion
Concentration of the ion on each side of the membrane

TABLE 5–6: The Resting Membrane Potential (E$_m$)

Inserting intracellular K$^+$ (145) and Na$^+$ (12) concentrations and extracellular K$^+$ (4.0) and Na$^+$ (140) concentrations into the *Goldman-Hodgkin-Katz equation* results in $E_m = -90$ mV
The cell interior is –90 mV, largely due to the movement of K$^+$ out of the cell via the Na$^+$-K$^+$ ATPase pump $$E_m = -61 \log \frac{3/2(140) + 0.01\,(12)}{3/2(4.0) + 0.01\,(145)} = -90\,\text{mv}$$
The E_m sets the stage for membrane depolarization and generation of the action potential; any change in plasma [K$^+$] alters action potential and cell excitability
Physiologic and pathologic factors affect K$^+$ distribution between ICF and ECF
Abbreviations: ICF, intracellular fluid; ECF, extracellular fluid

CELLULAR K$^+$ DISTRIBUTION

TABLE 5–7: Cellular K$^+$ Distribution
Maintenance of plasma K$^+$ homeostasis following a K$^+$ rich meal requires K$^+$ shift into cells
Cellular K$^+$ movement is the first response of the body
This is critical to prevent a lethal acute rise in plasma K$^+$ concentration as renal K$^+$ excretion requires several hours
Multiple physiologic and pathologic factors affect cellular K$^+$ distribution

TABLE 5–8: Factors Affecting Cellular K$^+$ Distribution

Insulin (secreted following a meal)

- K$^+$ concentration is maintained in the normal range by physiologic effects of insulin

  - Insulin moves K$^+$ into cells following a meal

  - Insulin stimulates K$^+$ uptake by increasing the activity and number of Na$^+$-K$^+$ ATPase pumps in the cell membrane

  - Intracellular K$^+$ shift is independent of glucose transport

  - Insulin deficiency (type 1 diabetic patients) is associated with hyperkalemia from impaired cellular K$^+$ uptake

Endogenous catecholamines (β_2 adrenergic)

- Promotes K$^+$ movement into cells (stimulation of Na$^+$-K$^+$ ATPase)

- Activation of β_2 receptors generates cyclic AMP and stimulates Na$^+$-K$^+$ ATPase to shift K$^+$ into cells

- Albuterol, a β_2 adrenergic agonist used for asthma lowers plasma [K$^+$] through increased cell uptake

- Propranolol, an antihypertensive medication, blocks β_2 adrenergic receptors and raises plasma [K$^+$]

- Digoxin intoxication raises plasma [K$^+$] by disrupting the Na$^+$-K$^+$ ATPase, thereby blocking cellular K$^+$ uptake

Exercise

- Exercise has a dual effect on cellular K$^+$ movement

  - A transient rise in plasma K$^+$ concentration occurs to increase blood flow to ischemic muscle

TABLE 5–8 (Continued)
■ Endogenous catecholamine secretion develops with exercise, moving K^+ back into the ICF (β_2 adrenergic receptors) and restores plasma K^+ concentration to normal
■ Level of exercise influences cellular K^+ release
■ Slow walking (0.3–0.4 mEq/L rise)
■ Moderate exercise (0.7–1.2 mEq/L rise
■ Point of exhaustion (2.0 mEq/L rise)
Change in pH (acidemia/alkalemia)
• Changes in pH are associated with cellular K^+ movement
■ Metabolic acidosis promotes K^+ exit from cells in exchange for protons (H^+) as the cells attempt to buffer the ECF pH
■ K^+ exchange for H^+ maintains electroneutrality across membranes
■ This effect occurs in nonanion gap metabolic acidoses rather than organic anion acidoses
■ In mineral metabolic acidosis, the anion Cl^- is unable to cross the membrane (K^+ must exit the cell to maintain electroneutrality)
■ In organic anion acidosis, the anion (lactate) crosses the membrane and K^+ is not required to exit the cell to maintain electroneutrality
■ Metabolic alkalosis causes an opposite effect

(continued)

TABLE 5–8 (Continued)

• Plasma [K⁺] increases/decreases by 0.4 mEq/L for every 0.1 unit decrease/increase in pH
■ There is wide variability (0.2–1.7 mEq/L for every 0.1 unit fall in pH) with pH change

Plasma osmolality

• Increased plasma osmolality (hyperglycemia) raises plasma [K⁺] as a result of a shift of K⁺ out of cells
■ K⁺ diffuses with water from the ICF into the ECF via solvent drag
■ Intracellular K⁺ concentration rises as water exits the cell, increasing K⁺ diffusion out of the cell
■ K⁺ concentration rises by 0.4–0.8 mEq/L per 10 mosm/kg increase in effective osmolality

Aldosterone

• Aldosterone may increase cellular K⁺ uptake, but its major effect is to enhance renal K⁺ excretion
Abbreviations: AMP, adenosine monophosphate; ICF, intracellular fluid, ECF, extracellular fluid

K+ HANDLING BY THE KIDNEY

TABLE 5–9: K+ Handling by the Kidney
Renal K+ handling occurs through glomerular filtration and both tubular reabsorption and secretion
Proximal tubule
100% of plasma K+ reaches the proximal tubule (freely filtered)
Proximal tubule reabsorbs 60–80% of filtered K+
K+ uptake occurs via passive mechanisms
• K+ is reabsorbed by a K+ transporter and through paracellular pathways coupled with Na+ and water
• Volume depletion increases Na+ and water reabsorption increasing K+ uptake
• Volume expansion inhibits passive diffusion of K+
Loop of Henle
K+ is both secreted and reabsorbed
Twenty-five percent of filtered K+ net is reabsorbed in this nephron segment
K+ enters the thin descending limb and at the tip of the loop of Henle reaches amounts that equal the original filtered load
In medullary thick ascending limb, K+ is actively and passively reabsorbed
• Active K+ transport occurs by the Na^+-K^+-$2Cl^-$ cotransporter, which is powered by Na^+-K^+ ATPase

(continued)

TABLE 5-9 (Continued)
Secondary active cotransport is driven by the steep Na$^+$ gradient across the apical membrane created by the ATPase
Medications such as loop diuretics and genetic disorders impair the activity of this cotransporter and result in Na$^+$ and K$^+$ wasting
Distal nephron
Approximately 10% of filtered K$^+$ reaches the distal tubule
K$^+$ secretion or reabsorption occurs in distal tubule, primarily in CCD
• High luminal Na$^+$ concentration and low luminal Cl$^-$ concentration stimulate K$^+$-Cl$^-$ cotransporter to secrete K$^+$
Abbreviation: CCD, cortical collecting duct

TABLE 5–10: Cell Types Involved in K$^+$ Transport in the Distal Nephron

Principal cell (see Figure 5–1)

Promotes K$^+$ secretion in the CCD

The apical membrane of this cell contains ENaC and K$^+$ channels, which act in concert with basolateral Na$^+$-K$^+$ ATPase to reabsorb Na$^+$ and secrete K$^+$

- Na$^+$ reabsorption through ENaC increases K$^+$ secretion by creating an electrochemical gradient for K$^+$ movement

- An electrical gradient develops because Na$^+$ leaves the lumen without an accompanying anion, creating a lumen negative charge that stimulates K$^+$ secretion

- Entry of Na$^+$ into cells increases basolateral Na$^+$-K$^+$ ATPase activity to lower intracellular Na$^+$

- Transporting three Na$^+$ ions out of the cell and two K$^+$ ions into the cell increases intracellular K$^+$ concentration and creates a gradient favoring K$^+$ exit through apical K$^+$ channels

Blockade of ENaC reduces renal K$^+$ excretion by blocking generation of the electrochemical gradient

Aldosterone receptor antagonists reduce apical ENaC function and Na$^+$-K$^+$ ATPase activity, limiting K$^+$ secretion

Alpha intercalated cell (see Figure 5–2)

This cell promotes K$^+$ reabsorption

- H$^+$-K$^+$ ATPase on the apical surface of this cell reabsorbs K$^+$ in exchange for H$^+$

Abbreviations: CCD, cortical collecting duct; ENaC, epithelial Na$^+$ channel

FIGURE 5–1: Principal cell in the CCD secretes K+ into urine via the passive K+ (ROMK) channel stimulated by the electrochemical gradient generated by Na+ reabsorption via the passive Na+ (ENaC) channel and action of the Na+-K+ ATPase enzyme on the basolateral membrane

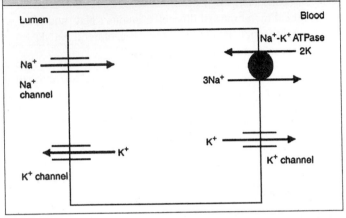

FIGURE 5–2: Alpha intercalated cell in the CCD reabsorbs K+ via the H+-K+ ATPase enzyme on the apical membrane and the action of the Na+-K+ ATPase enzyme on the basolateral membrane

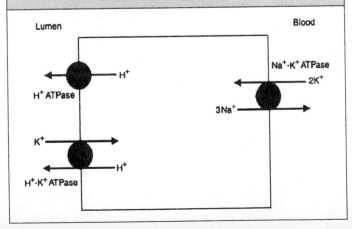

FACTORS CONTROLLING RENAL K^+ EXCRETION

TABLE 5–11: Factors That Influence Renal K^+ Excretion
Aldosterone
Plasma K^+ concentration
Tubular flow rate
Tubular Na^+ concentration
Antidiuretic hormone
Glucocorticoids
Metabolic alkalosis
Metabolic acidosis
Impermeant anions in urine (sulfate, bicarbonate, carbenicillin)

TABLE 5–12: Four Major Factors that Control Renal K⁺ Excretion

Aldosterone

- Binds the mineralocorticoid receptor

- Stimulates Na^+ entry (ENaC) and enhances basolateral Na^+-K^+ ATPase activity

- This creates an *electrical potential* for K^+ secretion (lumen negative charge for K^+ movement), and *diffusional gradient* for K^+ secretion (raising intracellular K^+ concentration)

Plasma K^+ concentration

- Plasma K^+ concentration > 5.0 mEq/L produces effects on the principal cell that are similar to aldosterone

- This represents a protective mechanism to maintain renal K^+ excretion even when aldosterone is deficient or absent

Urine flow rate and Na^+ delivery

- These factors act on the luminal side (urinary space) to modify K^+ excretion

- High urine flow rates enhance K^+ secretion by maintaining low urine [K^+] and a favorable diffusional gradient

- Urinary Na^+ delivery to the principal cell promotes K^+ secretion by enhancing Na^+ entry (ENaC), creating a favorable electrochemical gradient

Abbreviation: ENaC, epithelial Na^+ channel

HYPOKALEMIA

Hypokalemia is defined as plasma K$^+$ concentration
< 3.5 mEq/L

ETIOLOGY

TABLE 5–13: General Categories of Causes of Hypokalemia
Dietary K$^+$
• Inadequate oral intake (in combination with other factors)
Cellular K$^+$ uptake
• Insulin
• Catecholamines (B_2 adrenergic)
• Metabolic alkalosis
• Hypokalemic periodic paralysis
• Cell growth from B12 therapy
• Cesium chloride, barium intoxication, risperidone, quetiapine, and chloroquine
Renal K$^+$ excretion
• Aldosteronism (primary or secondary)
• Corticosteroid excess
• High urine flow rate from diuretics
• High distal Na$^+$ delivery
• Renal tubular acidosis

(continued)

TABLE 5–13 (Continued)
• Drugs
■ Amphotericin B
■ Diuretics
■ Aminoglycosides
■ Lithium
■ Cisplatinum
■ Some penicillins
• Genetic renal diseases
■ Bartter syndrome
■ Gitelman's syndrome
■ Liddle's syndrome
■ Apparent mineralocorticoid excess
Gastrointestinal K⁺ loss
• Vomiting
• Diarrhea, ostomy losses
Skin K⁺ loss
• Strenuous exercise
• Severe heat stress

TABLE 5–14: Increased Cellular K+ Uptake
Exogenous insulin administration shifts K+ into cells
• Diabetic patients given insulin develop hypokalemia due to cellular K+ uptake
β_2 adrenergic agonists mediate cell uptake by β_2 receptors
• β_2 adrenergic agonist therapy in the patient with severe asthma (albuterol) or in labor (ritodrine) causes hypokalemia through cell shift
Metabolic alkalosis promotes cell K+ shift
• This acid-base disorder is precipitated by vomiting and diuretic use, which contributes to renal K+ losses
Hypokalemic periodic paralysis causes hypokalemia from cellular K+ uptake precipitated by a carbohydrate meal
Rapid synthesis of red blood cells induced by B_{12} or iron therapy may cause hypokalemia as new cells utilize K+

TABLE 5–15: Increased Renal K$^+$ Excretion

Medications increase renal K$^+$ excretion in various nephron segments

In PCT

- Acetazolamide blocks carbonic anhydrase and induces bicarbonaturia and K$^+$ wasting

- Osmotic diuretics increase flow through PCT, reducing Na$^+$, water and K$^+$ reabsorption

- Aminoglycosides and cisplatin injure PCT cells and cause K$^+$ wasting

In TALH

- Na$^+$-K$^+$-2Cl$^-$ transporter reabsorbs K$^+$ in TALH

- Loop diuretics inhibit function of this transporter and reduce K$^+$ reabsorption via paracellular and transcellular pathways

In DCT

- Thiazide diuretics block the NCC in DCT, increasing Na$^+$ delivery and urine to principal cells in CCD

- Fludrocortisone binds the aldosterone receptor and stimulates renal K$^+$ secretion in principal cells

- Amphotericin B disrupts principal cell membranes, allowing K$^+$ to leak out of the cell

Clinical disease states increase renal K$^+$ excretion

Primary or secondary aldosteronism and corticosteroid excess induce hypokalemia by stimulation of mineralocorticoid receptors and K$^+$ secretion in CCD

TABLE 5–15 (Continued)

Primary or acquired forms of RTA cause hypokalemia through tubular dysfunction proximally (type 2 RTA) or distally (type 1 RTA)

Inherited renal disorders cause K⁺ wasting and hypokalemia

- In TALH, various mutations cause cellular dysfunction, resulting in Bartter syndrome (see Table 7–16)

- Mutation of the gene encoding the thiazide sensitive NCC causes Gitelman's syndrome (see Table 7–16)

- Activating mutations in subunits of the ENaC (β, γ) cause Liddle's syndrome (see Table 7–15)

Abbreviations: PCT, proximal convoluted tubule; TALH, thick ascending limb of Henle; DCT, distal tubule; NCC, Na⁺-Cl⁻ cotransporter; CCD, cortical collecting duct; RTA, renal tubular acidosis; ENaC, epithelial Na⁺ channel

TABLE 5–16: Other Sources of K⁺ Loss from the Body

GI K⁺ losses

- Vomiting, diarrhea, and excessive ostomy output may cause excessive K⁺ losses from the GI tract

Skin K⁺ losses

- Extreme heat (hyperthermia) or severe exercise causes hypokalemia

Abbreviation: GI, gastrointestinal

APPROACH TO THE PATIENT

TABLE 5–17: Approach to the Patient with Hypokalemia
A stepwise approach to hypokalemia assures accurate diagnosis
The initial evaluation of hypokalemia divides pseudohypokalemia from true hypokalemia, followed by separating cell shift of potassium from excessive renal or GI losses of K$^+$ (see Figure 5–3)
Step 1 Exclude pseudohypokalemia and cell shift
Step 2 Measure the patient's *blood pressure* • *Hypertension* associated with hypokalemia is then classified based on concentrations of *renin* and *aldosterone* High versus low renin High versus low aldosterone • *Hypotension* or *normotension* associated with hypokalemia requires measurement of urinary K$^+$ concentration   ▪ Renal versus extrarenal causes
Step 3 Measure *acid-base status* to determine further classification of hypokalemia with normal or low blood pressure • Metabolic acidosis • Metabolic alkalosis
Abbreviation: GI, gastrointestinal

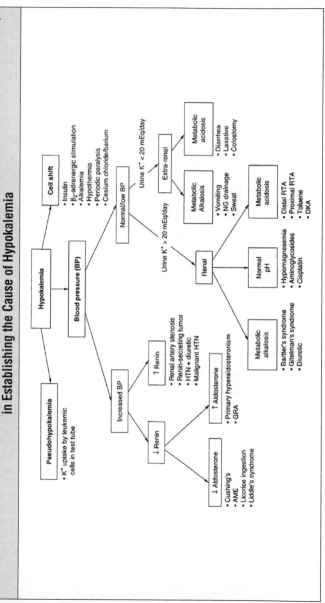

FIGURE 5–3: Diagram of Approach to Hypokalemia Emphasizing Utility of Blood Pressure, Plasma Renin Activity and Aldosterone Concentration, and Acid-Base Status (Metabolic Acidosis vs. Metabolic Alkalosis) in Establishing the Cause of Hypokalemia

CLINICAL MANIFESTATIONS

TABLE 5–18: Clinical Manifestations of Hypokalemia
Clinical manifestations are effects of serum K+ deficits on action potential generation in excitable tissues
Impaired neuromuscular function precipitates a spectrum of findings ranging from muscle weakness to frank paralysis
Cardiac disturbances
• Various atrial and ventricular arrhythmias
• Hypokalemic arrhythmias may be fatal in patients on digoxin or in those with underlying cardiac disease
• Abnormal myocardial contractile function
Renal manifestations
• Impaired urinary concentration (polyuria)
• Increased renal ammonia production and bicarbonate reabsorption (perpetuating metabolic alkalosis)
• Renal dysfunction from either tubular vacuolization (hypokalemic nephropathy) or myoglobinuria
Metabolic perturbations
• Hyperglycemia from decreased insulin release
• Impaired hepatic glycogen and protein synthesis
Other organ systems
• Respiratory failure from diaphragmatic muscle weakness
• Ileus from reduced smooth muscle contractility

TREATMENT

TABLE 5–19: Treatment of Hypokalemia
Treatment of hypokalemia is guided by two major factors
Determine physiologic effects
Physiologic effects of hypokalemia are best judged by:
• Physical examination of neuromuscular function
■ Muscle weakness is present with hypokalemia, while paralysis signals severe hypokalemia
• ECG interrogation of the cardiac conduction system
■ Prominent U waves (see Figure 5–4) suggest a serum K$^+$ concentration in the 1.5–2.0 mEq/L range
Approximate the K$^+$ deficit
K$^+$ deficit is approximated by the following:
• Underlying mechanism of hypokalemia
■ Less with cell shift, more with renal/GI losses
• The prevailing serum K$^+$ concentration
■ 3.0–3.5 mEq/L range, total body K$^+$ deficits reach 200–400 mEq
■ 2.0–3.0 mEq/L range, total body K$^+$ deficits reach 400–800 mEq
Abbreviations: ECG, electrocardiography; GI, gastrointestinal

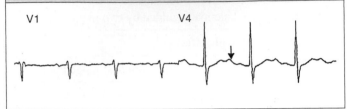

FIGURE 5–4: Electrocardiogram of Hypokalemia Demonstrating the U Wave (Arrow) Indicative of Severe Hypokalemia

TABLE 5–20: Correction of Hypokalemia
Oral KCl (40–80 mEq/day) is preferred with mild to moderate deficits (2.5–3.5 mEq/L)
IV KCl (20–40 mEq/L in 1 L of 0.45 normal saline at a rate ≤ 20 mEq/h) plus oral KCl are required for severe K⁺ deficits (< 2.5 mEq/L)
• Faster rates are avoided as they injure veins (sclerosis) and cause cardiac dysrrhythmias
Correction of the cause of hypokalemia is part of therapy
Abbreviation: IV, intravenous

HYPERKALEMIA

Hyperkalemia is defined as plasma K⁺ concentration > 5.5 mEq/L.

ETIOLOGY

TABLE 5–21: Basics of Hyperkalemia
Hyperkalemia is broken down into the following:
• Pseudohyperkalemia
• True hyperkalemia
■ Impaired cell K$^+$ uptake
■ Decreased renal K$^+$ excretion

TABLE 5–22: Causes of Pseudohyperkalemia
Pseudohyperkalemia rarely falsely elevates the serum K$^+$ concentration
• K$^+$ release from cells within the test tube
• Cell lysis following prolonged tourniquet application
• K$^+$ release from large cell numbers (white blood cells >100,000/mm^3; platelets >1,000,000/mm^3)

TABLE 5–23: Causes of True Hyperkalemia
Dietary K$^+$
• Excessive oral or IV intake (in combination with other factors)
Cellular K$^+$ release/impaired cellular uptake
• Lack of insulin (fasting, diabetes mellitus)
• β_2 adrenergic blockade
• Metabolic acidosis
• Hyperkalemic periodic paralysis
• Succinylcholine
• Hyperosmolality (hyperglycemia, mannitol)
• Digoxin toxicity
• Cell lysis (hemolysis, rhabdomyolysis, tumor lysis)
• Severe exercise
Renal K$^+$ retention
• Hypoaldosteronism (see Table 6–43)
▪ Hypoadrenalism (Addison's disease)
▪ Hyporeninemic hypoaldosteronism
▪ Heparin
▪ ACE-inhibitors, angiotensin receptor blockers
▪ NSAIDs, selective COX-2 inhibitors

TABLE 5–23 (Continued)
• Low urine flow rate and/or decreased distal Na$^+$ delivery
• Renal tubular resistance to aldosterone
■ Obstructive uropathy
■ Systemic lupus erythematosus
■ Sickle cell disease
• Drugs
• Genetic renal diseases
■ Gordon's syndrome (pseudohypoaldosteronism type-2)
• Advanced chronic kidney disease or acute kidney injury
Abbreviations: IV, intravenous; NSAIDs, nonsteroidal anti-inflammatory drugs; COX, cyclooxygenase

TABLE 5–24: Impaired Cellular K+ Uptake

Deficient endogenous or exogenous insulin reduces K^+ entry into cells and causes hyperkalemia

- Patients with insulin-dependent diabetes mellitus

Therapy with β_2 adrenergic antagonists raises serum K^+ concentration through inhibition of cellular K^+ uptake

- Treatment of hypertension and heart disease with propranolol, labetalol, or carvedilol

Nonanion gap (mineral) metabolic acidosis promotes K^+ shift out of cells and hyperkalemia

Hyperkalemic periodic paralysis impairs cellular K^+ uptake and causes hyperkalemia

Hyperosmolality shifts K^+ out of cells via solvent drag and elevates serum K^+ concentration

- Diabetes mellitus with hyperglycemia

- Hyperosmolar substances (mannitol, dextran, HES)

Release of K^+ from cells causes hyperkalemia

- Lysis of red blood cells (hemolysis), muscle cells (rhabdomyolysis), and tumor cells (tumor lysis)

Abbreviation: HES, hydroxyethyl starch

TABLE 5–25: Decreased Renal K$^+$ Secretion

Medications reduce renal K$^+$ excretion by blunting the kaliuretic mechanisms of the principal cell

- Reduce aldosterone synthesis
  - Nonsteroidal anti-inflammatory drugs, ACE inhibitors, angiotensin receptor antagonists, and heparin
- Block aldosterone effect
  - Spironolactone and eplerenone
- Block ENaC on principal cell
  - Amiloride, triamterene, trimethoprim and pentamidine
- Inhibition of Na$^+$-K$^+$ ATPase
  - Digoxin, cyclosporine and tacrolimus

Clinical disease states reduce renal K$^+$ excretion

- Reduced functioning nephron number
  - Advanced chronic kidney disease or acute kidney injury
- Aldosterone deficiency
  - Adrenal dysfunction, diabetes mellitus, and other forms of hyporeninemic hypoaldosteronism
- Tubular resistance to aldosterone or defects in tubular K$^+$ secretion
  - Obstructive uropathy, SLE, and sickle cell nephropathy
- Inherited disorders
  - Pseudohypoaldosteronism types 1 and 2

(continued)

TABLE 5–25 (Continued)
• Reduced distal Na$^+$ delivery and urine flow rate
■ True volume depletion (nausea, vomiting, diarrhea, diuretics) and effective volume depletion (CHF, cirrhosis, nephrotic syndrome)
Abbreviations: ACE, angiotensin converting enzyme; ENaC, epithelial Na$^+$ channel; SLE, systemic lupus erythematosus; CHF, congestive heart failure

TABLE 5–26: Approach to the Patient with Hyperkalemia

- The patient with hyperkalemia should be evaluated in a stepwise fashion to distinguish pseudohyperkalemia from true hyperkalemia, and then cellular shift from a renal K^+ excretory deficit (see Figure 5–5)

Step 1 Exclude *pseudohyperkalemia* and *cellular K⁺ shift*

Step 2 Measure *urinary K⁺ excretion* and calculate the TTKG and/or FEK
- TTKG provides a more accurate assessment of the tubular fluid K^+ concentration at the end of the cortical collecting tubule
  - Defect in renal K^+ excretion or another process
- TTKG is calculated by measuring urinary and serum K^+ and osmolality (osm), respectively and inserting the values into the formula
- In order to calculate the TTKG the urine $[Na^+]$ must be greater than as equal to 20 mEg/L and the urine osmolality must be greater than serum osmolality

$$\textbf{TTKG} = \text{Urine } [K^+] \div (\text{urine osm/plasma osm}) \div \text{serum } [K^+]$$

Step 3 Assess *urinary K⁺ excretion* and *TTKG* data
- Reduced urine K^+ excretion and a TTKG < 5 suggest a renal defect in K^+ excretion
  - Measure and classify patient based on plasma *aldosterone* and *renin* concentrations
    - Normal versus low aldosterone
    - Low aldosterone with either high or low renin
- Elevated K^+ excretion and TTKG > 5 are categorized as a nonrenal cause of hyperkalemia
  - Diet, drugs, or internal factors

Abbreviations: TTKG, transtubular K^+ gradient; FEK, fractional excretion of K^+

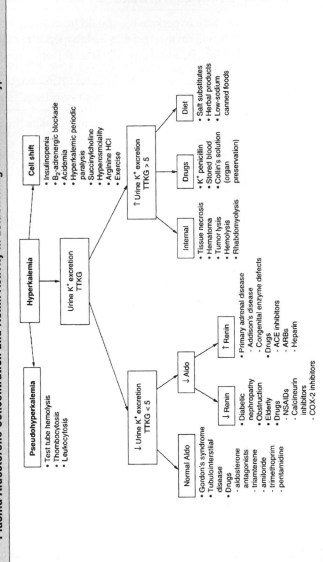

FIGURE 5–5: Diagram of Approach to Hyperkalemia Emphasizing Utility of Urine K⁺ Excretion, as well as Plasma Aldosterone Concentration and Renin Activity in Establishing the Cause of Hyperkalemia

CLINICAL MANIFESTATIONS

TABLE 5–27: Clinical Manifestations of Hyperkalemia
Clinical manifestations of hyperkalemia are due to pathologic effects of high serum K$^+$ concentration on generation of action potentials in excitable tissues (heart and neuromuscular tissues)
Various degrees of muscle weakness and paralysis
Respiratory failure from diaphragmatic muscle weakness
Cardiac disturbances
• Various AV nodal blocks, ventricular arrhythmias, and asystole
• Abnormal myocardial contractile function causing hypotension
Abbreviation: AV, antrioventricular

TREATMENT

TABLE 5–28: Factors Guiding Therapy of Hyperkalemia
Hyperkalemia is potentially lethal and must be promptly treated
The physiologic effects of hyperkalemia:
• Signs of neuromuscular dysfunction include variable muscle weakness
• ECG evidence of cardiac conduction disturbances
■ Earliest is tenting of the T waves
■ QRS complex widens and P wave disappears (see Figure 5–6)
■ Last are sine wave pattern, AV block and ventricular fibrillation or asystole
The underlying cause of hyperkalemia
• Differentiate cell shift versus impaired renal excretion
Abbreviations: ECG, electrocardiogram; AV, atrioventricular

FIGURE 5–6: Electrocardiogram of Hyperkalemia Demonstrating Loss of P Waves, Development of Peaked T Waves, and Widened QRS Complexes Indicative of Severe Hyperkalemia

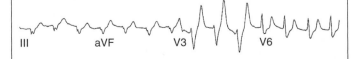

TABLE 5–29: Steps in the Treatment of Hyperkalemia

Rapid therapy is required to prevent fatal outcomes

Stabilization of excitable membranes (cardiac tissues)

- IV Ca^{2+} under cardiac monitoring; Ca^{2+} should be given as a slower drip to patients on digoxin

Shift K$^+$ into cells

- Intravenous regular insulin with glucose in nondiabetic patients

  - Lowers serum K$^+$ concentration (0.5–1.0 mEq/L)

- High dose β_2 adrenergic agonists

  - Lowers serum K$^+$ concentration (0.6–1.0 mEq/L)

- Combine insulin and β_2 adrenergic agonists

- Na$^+$ bicarbonate in patients with a nonanion gap metabolic acidosis and can tolerate an Na$^+$ load

  - Minimal effect (less effective other choices)

Remove K$^+$ from the body

- Increase gastrointestinal K$^+$ excretion

  - Cation-exchange resin (Na$^+$ polystyrene with sorbitol) as oral preparation or retention enema

- Enhance renal K$^+$ excretion

  - High dose loop diuretics

- Hemodialysis quickly removes K$^+$ from the body

(continued)

TABLE 5–29 (Continued)
Additional measures to treat hyperkalemia
• Correct the primary cause of hyperkalemia
• Appropriately adjust dietary K$^+$ intake for level of kidney function
Abbreviation: IV, intravenous

TABLE 5–30: Clinical Treatment of Hyperkalemia				
Treatment	**Dose**	**Onset**	**Time**	**Mechanism**
Ca gluconate (10%)	10–20 mL IV	1–5 min	30–60 min	Stabilize membranes
Insulin and glucose	10–20 U of IV insulin and 25 g of glucose	30 min	4–6 h	Cell uptake
Albuterol (β_2-agonist)	20 mg in 4 mL normal saline in nebulizer	30 min	1–2 h	Cell uptake
Terbutaline (β_2-agonist)	0.7 mg/kg SQ	20–30 min	1–2 h	Cell uptake
Na bicarbonate	50–75 mEq IV	5–10 min	2–12 h	Cell uptake
Na polystyrene sulfonate	30–45 g oral 50–100 g enema	2–4 h	4–12 h	GI excretion
Hemodialysis	1–2 mEq/L K bath	—	2–8 h	Removal
Abbreviations: IV, intravenous; U, units; GI, gastrointestinal; SQ, subcutaneous				

6
Metabolic Acidosis

ACID-BASE CHEMISTRY AND BIOLOGY

TABLE 6–1: General Principles of Acid-Base Homeostasis
Acid-base homeostasis consists of the precise regulation of CO_2 tension by the respiratory system and plasma bicarbonate (HCO_3^-) concentration [HCO_3^-] by the kidney
The kidney regulates plasma [HCO_3^-] by altering HCO_3^- reabsorption and eliminating protons (H^+)
Body fluid pH is determined by CO_2 tension and [HCO_3^-]
Body fluids can generally be readily sampled and analyzed with a blood gas instrument that determines CO_2 tension (in arterial blood, $PaCO_2$), pH, and [HCO_3^-], the latter is generally calculated
Primary abnormalities of CO_2 tension are considered respiratory disturbances, whereas primary derangements of [HCO_3^-] are metabolic disturbances

TABLE 6–2: Buffering

Bronsted-Lowry definition

An acid is a chemical that donates a H^+, and a base is a H^+ acceptor

For an acid (HA) and its conjugate base (A^-), we describe its strength (or tendency to donate a H^+) by its dissociation constant K_{eq} shown in Eq. (6-1)

Buffering describes the capacity of a solution to resist pH change when a strong (i.e., highly dissociated) acid or alkali is added

In mammals the most important buffer in the extracellular space is the bicarbonate buffer system (capacity: bicarbonate- 375 mmol; phosphate < 15 mmol; protein < 10 mmol); inorganic phosphate and proteins are less important; hemoglobin contributes 80% of the protein buffering capacity and most of the remaining 20% is carried out by albumin

In the intracellular space proteins are quantitatively the most important buffer followed by bicarbonate and intracellular phosphate (capacity: proteins- 400 mmol; bicarbonate- 330 mmol; phosphate- < 50 mmol)

While cytosolic or intracellular pH (pHi) is more important in predicting physiologic and clinical consequences than extracellular pH, it is difficult to measure in vivo; because extracellular acid-base status is still informative, and can be measured, we focus our clinical efforts on this information

Lewis definition (Figure 6–2)

An acid is a chemical that is an electron-pair acceptor, and a base is an electron-pair donor

TABLE 6–2 (Continued)

When a substance is metabolized to something more anionic-H^+s are generated

- When a neutral substrate is metabolized to an anion proton(s) are generated (example: glucose to lactate); when a cation is metabolized to a neutral substance proton(s) are generated (cationic amino acids)

When a substance is metabolized to something more cationic-H^+s are consumed and bicarbonate generated

- When a neutral substrate is metabolized to a cation proton(s) are consumed; when an anion is metabolized to a neutral substance proton(s) are consumed and a bicarbonate generated (citrate or anionic amino acids)

$$[HA] = K_{eq} \times [H^+][A^-] \tag{6-1}$$

After rearranging and log transformation

$$pH = pK + \log_{10} \frac{[A^-]}{[HA]} \tag{6-2}$$

FIGURE 6–1: Buffering in the Intracellular and Extracellular Spaces

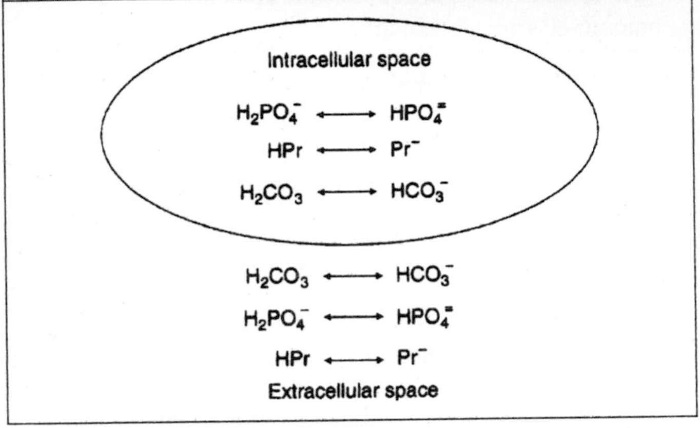

Intracellular space

$H_2PO_4^- \longleftrightarrow HPO_4^=$

$HPr \longleftrightarrow Pr^-$

$H_2CO_3 \longleftrightarrow HCO_3^-$

$H_2CO_3 \longleftrightarrow HCO_3^-$

$H_2PO_4^- \longleftrightarrow HPO_4^=$

$HPr \longleftrightarrow Pr^-$

Extracellular space

TABLE 6–3: The Bicarbonate Buffering System

It is generally assumed that equilibrium conditions apply to the bicarbonate buffer system in blood because of the abundance of carbonic anhydrase (CA) in red cells and the high permeability of the red cell membrane to components of the bicarbonate buffer system. Therefore, we can express the following equations:

$$H^+ + HCO_3 \xrightarrow{K_{eq}} H_2CO_3 \qquad (6\text{-}3)$$

Or

$$[H^+] = K_{eq} \times \frac{[H_2CO_3]}{[HCO_3^-]} \qquad (6\text{-}4)$$

Furthermore, H_2CO_3 is defined by the partial pressure of CO_2 and the solubility of CO_2 in physiologic fluids that is, for all intents and purposes, a constant S. We can, therefore, rearrange Eq. (6-4) to read

$$[H^+] = K \times \frac{S \times PCO_2}{[HCO_3^-]} \qquad (6\text{-}5)$$

Taking the antilog of both sides we get

$$\mathbf{pH} = pK + \log_{10} \frac{HCO_3^-}{S \times PCO_2} \qquad (6\text{-}6)$$

This is called the *Henderson-Hasselbalch* equation. In blood (at 37°C), the pK referred to in Eq. (6-6) is 6.1 and the solubility coefficient for CO_2 (S) is 0.03. Therefore, we can simplify this expression to

$$\mathbf{pH} = 6.1 + \log_{10} \frac{[HCO_3^-]}{0.03 \times PaCO_2} \qquad (6\text{-}7)$$

This formula allows us to view acid-base disorders as being attributable to the numerator of the ratio (metabolic processes), the denominator (respiratory processes), or both (mixed or complex acid-base disorders)

TABLE 6–4: Assessing Acid-Base Balance

Because of the importance of the bicarbonate buffer system in overall acid-base homeostasis, we generally consider the addition of a proton as equivalent to a decrease in total body HCO_3^- and loss of a proton as a gain in HCO_3^-

The classic normal values for an arterial blood gas are pH: 7.4; $[HCO_3^-]$: 24 mEq/L; and $PaCO_2$: 40 mmHg

The kidneys regulate serum $[HCO_3^-]$ and acid-base balance by reclaiming filtered HCO_3^- and generating new HCO_3^- to replace that lost internally in titrating metabolic acid and externally (e.g., from the gastrointestinal tract)

Approximately 1 mmol of H^+/kg body weight per day is generated from the metabolism of nonvolatile acids and bases and the ingestion of a normal "Western diet" to maintain acid-base homeostasis the kidney must excrete this acid load

The role of the kidney in acid-base homeostasis can be divided into two basic functions: (1) the reabsorption of filtered bicarbonate and (2) the excretion of the acid load derived from dietary metabolism

FIGURE 6–2: Many Reactions Involve the Loss or Gain of Protons. To understand whether acid or base is produced one simply examines the initial substrates and final products. To do this, it is helpful to think of acids and bases as "lewis" acids and bases; in other words, to consider acids as electron acceptors rather than as proton donors. In concrete terms, when a substrate is metabolized to something more anionic (e.g., glucose is metabolized to lactate), a H^+ is generated. Conversely, if a substrate is metabolized to something more cationic (e.g., lactate is metabolized to CO_2 and H_2O via the tricarboxylic acid [TCA] cycle), a H^+ is consumed

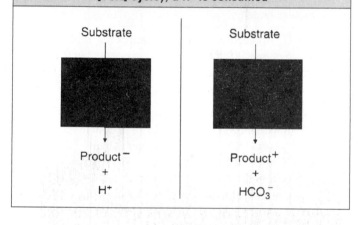

ACID EXCRETION BY THE KIDNEY

<table>
<tr><td colspan="1">

TABLE 6–5: Assessing Acid-Base Balance—Bicarbonate Reclamation

</td></tr>
<tr><td>

Regarding overall acid-base handling by the kidney, there is a strong relationship between acid secretion and reclamation of filtered bicarbonate, as well as the production of new bicarbonate in the distal nephron

</td></tr>
<tr><td>

Bicarbonate reclamation

</td></tr>
<tr><td>

First, plasma is filtered at the glomerulus and HCO_3^- enters the tubular lumen

</td></tr>
<tr><td>

Each HCO_3^- molecule reclaimed requires the epithelial secretion of one H^+; this H^+ secretion occurs via the Na^+-H^+ exchanger on the luminal membrane or through an electrogenic H^+ ATPase

</td></tr>
<tr><td>

We can think of the HCO_3^- reabsorption processes establishing a *plasma threshold* for bicarbonate, i.e., that level of plasma HCO_3^- at which measurable HCO_3^- appears in urine; we can also define the maximal net activity of tubular HCO_3^- reabsorption as the T_{max}; the T_{max} and *plasma threshold* for HCO_3^- are intimately related; as the T_{max} for HCO_3^- increases, the *plasma threshold* for HCO_3^- increases, and vice versa

</td></tr>
<tr><td>

HCO_3^- reclamation involves a considerable amount of H^+ secretion by the tubules

</td></tr>
<tr><td>

Bicarbonate reclamation is closely related to Na^+ reabsorption and is, therefore, sensitive to a number of other influences that impact Na^+ reabsorption

</td></tr>
</table>

TABLE 6–5 (Continued)

- States of ECF volume expansion and decreases in PCO_2 decrease the apparent T_{max} for HCO_3^-, whereas ECF volume contraction and increases in PCO_2 increase the apparent T_{max} for HCO_3^-

- Parathyroid hormone inhibits proximal tubule HCO_3^- reabsorption and lowers the apparent T_{max} and plasma threshold for HCO_3^-

- The majority of HCO_3^- reabsorption (approximately 80–90%) takes place in proximal tubule

- The enzyme carbonic anhydrase is expressed intracellularly (type II isoform), as well as on the luminal membrane of the proximal tubule cell (type IV isoform), which allows the secreted H^+ to combine with tubular fluid HCO_3^- to form H_2CO_3; this H_2CO_3 rapidly dissociates to form H_2O and CO_2, which then can reenter the proximal tubule cell

- Intracellularly, water dissociates into H^+ and OH^-; intracellular carbonic anhydrase catalyzes the formation of HCO_3^- from CO_2 and OH^-; bicarbonate leaves the cell via several bicarbonate transport proteins including the Na^+-bicarbonate cotransporter, as well as the Cl^--HCO_3^- exchanger

- In proximal tubule, where the reclamation of filtered HCO_3^- from the blood occurs, HCO_3^- is formed inside renal tubular cells when either H^+ secretion or ammonium (NH_4^+) synthesis occurs; the HCO_3^- is then transported back into blood predominantly via the basolateral Na^+-$3HCO_3^-$ cotransporter

Abbreviation: ECF, extracellular fluid

TABLE 6–6: Assessing Acid-Base Balance—Distal Nephron

Production of new bicarbonate by the distal nephron

Proton secretion by distal nephron is aided by the production of an electrogenic gradient. Protons are secreted by alpha intercalated cells

The gradient is produced by Na^+ removal from the luminal fluid in excess of anion reabsorption, this favors H^+ secretion; there is also direct pumping of H^+ into the tubular lumen

Na^+-H^+ exchange, as well as the activities of the vacuolar H^+ ATPase and the Na^+-K^+ ATPase in intercalated and principal cells accomplish these tasks

Cl^- exchange with bicarbonate on the basolateral side of these distal tubular cells allows for proton secretion to be translated into bicarbonate addition to blood

The epithelial membrane in the distal nephron must not allow back leak of H^+ or loss of the electrogenic gradient

Under normal circumstances, urine pH can be as low as 4.4; this represents a 1000:1 gradient of $[H^+]$ between tubular fluid and ECF

Abbreviation: ECF, extracellular fluid

TABLE 6–7: Net Acid Excretion

NAE is the total amount of H^+ excreted by the kidneys; quantitatively, we can calculate NAE to be the amount of H^+ (both buffered and free) excreted in urine minus the amount of HCO_3^- that failed to be reclaimed and was lost in urine. Some authors also subtract the urinary loss of other anions that have the potential of being converted in the body to bicarbonate (largely citrate)

Because H^+ secretion into the tubule lumen results in a 1:1 HCO_3^- addition to the ECF, NAE equals the amount of new HCO_3^- generated

NAE is accomplished through two processes that are historically separated on the basis of a colorimetric indicator (phenolphthalein) that detects pH changes effectively between pH 5 and 8; that acid, which can be detected by titrating sufficient alkali into urine to achieve color changes with this indicator is called titratable acid, and is mostly phosphate in the monobasic ($H_2PO_4^-$) form

Nontitratable acid excretion occurs primarily in the form of NH_4^+; this is not detected by phenolphthalein since the pK (approximately 9.2) for ammonium is too high

The majority of NAE is in the form of protons bound to buffers, either phosphate or ammonium; this makes it possible to elaborate a much less acid urine but still achieve adequate NAE

Even though most clinicians equate NAE with an acidic urine, it is important to recognize that a low urine pH does not necessarily mean increased NAE; for example, at a urine pH of 4.0 the free H^+ concentration is only 0.1 mmol; in a 70-kg person on an average Western diet one can see that free protons would make up only a small fraction of the approximately 70 mmol of net acid excreted daily

(continued)

TABLE 6–7 (Continued)

There are several pathologic conditions (discussed later) in which the urine pH is relatively acid but NAE is insufficient

In subjects that consume a typical Western diet, adequate NAE occurs through the functions of both the proximal tubule to synthesize NH_4^+ (which generates HCO_3^-) and distal and collecting tubules where H^+ secretion occurs

NAE is influenced by several factors including the serum K^+ concentration (serum K^+ elevations decrease NH_4^+ excretion, while decreases enhance distal nephron H^+ secretion), $PaCO_2$, and the effects of aldosterone

Quantitatively, NAE is usually evenly divided between titratable acid and ammonium excretion however, our capacity to increase NAE is mostly dependent on enhanced ammoniagenesis and NH_4^+ excretion

Abbreviations: NAE, net acid excretion; ECF, extracellular fluid

TABLE 6–8: Ammoniagenesis

The older view that NH_4^+ excretion was accomplished by simple passive trapping of NH_4^+ in the tubular lumen has been revised; we now understand that the excretion of NH_4^+ is more *active*

First, in proximal tubule cells, there is deamination of glutamine to form α-KG and two NH_4^+ via the sequential action of glutaminase and glutamate dehydrogenase. The further metabolism of α-KG to CO_2 and H_2O generates two new HCO_3^- molecules as discussed earlier; proximal tubule cells actively secrete NH_4^+ into the lumen, probably via the luminal Na^+-H^+ exchanger; NH_4^+ can substitute for H^+ and be transported into the urine in exchange for Na^+

NH_4^+ is subsequently reabsorbed in the medullary thick ascending limb of Henle where it can be transported instead of K^+ via the Na^+-K^+-$2Cl^-$ cotransporter; this increases medullary interstitial concentrations of NH_4^+

Interstitial NH_4^+ enters the collecting duct cell, substituting for K^+ on the basolateral Na^+-K^+ ATPase; the NH_4^+ is next secreted into the tubular lumen, possibly by substitution for H^+ in the apical Na^+-H^+ exchanger or H^+-K^+ ATPase and is ultimately excreted into the final urine

It is important to note that the net generation of any HCO_3^- from α-KG metabolism is dependent on this excretion of NH_4^+; if this NH_4^+ molecule is not excreted in urine, it is returned via the systemic circulation to the liver, where it will be used to form urea at the expense of generating two H^+s; in this case, the HCO_3^- molecules generated by the metabolism of α-KG are neutralized and no net HCO_3^- generation results

(continued)

TABLE 6–8 (Continued)

Because routine clinical measurement of urinary NH_4^+ concentrations never became standard, our appreciation of NH_4^+ in net acid-base balance during pathophysiologic conditions was delayed until recently; urinary $[NH_4^+]$ is estimated by calculations based on urinary electrolyte concentrations (either urinary anion gap or urinary osmolar gap) that are routinely measured

Abbreviation: α-KG, alpha-ketoglutarate

TABLE 6–9: Clinical Approach to the Patient with an Acid-Base Disorder

The information necessary to approach a suspected acid-base disorder involves a blood gas (which gives pH, PaO_2, $PaCO_2$, and calculated $[HCO_3^-]$ values) and serum chemistry panel (which gives serum Na^+, K^+, Cl^-, and total CO_2 content); the total CO_2 content (TCO_2), which is the sum of the serum $[HCO_3^-]$ and dissolved CO_2 (usually determined on a venous serum sample) is often referred to as the "CO_2"; however, it must not be confused with the $PaCO_2$, which refers to the partial pressure of CO_2 in arterial blood. Since the serum $[HCO_3^-]$ or TCO_2 includes a component of dissolved CO_2, it is often 1–2 mEq/L higher than the calculated $[HCO_3^-]$ derived from arterial blood gases. Some laboratory reports refer to total CO_2 content as serum bicarbonate. Although there is a difference between the two values, it is often not clinically significant

Eight Steps to Evaluating a Suspected Acid-Base Disturbance

Step 1 Verify that the blood gas values are correct using either the Henderson-Hasselbalch equation or the Henderson equation

- In order to use the Henderson equation one must convert pH to $[H^+]$ (see Table 6–10)

Step 2 What is the blood pH (is the patient acidemic or alkalemic)?

- Based on a normal sea level pH of 7.4 ± 0.02, a significant decrease in pH or acidemia means that the primary ongoing process is an acidosis; conversely, an increase in pH or alkalemia indicates that the primary ongoing process is an alkalosis

(continued)

TABLE 6–9 (Continued)

Step 3 Identify the primary disturbance

- In order to accomplish this one must examine the directional changes of $PaCO_2$ and serum $[HCO_3^-]$ from normal

- If pH is low and $[HCO_3^-]$ is low, then metabolic acidosis is the primary disturbance

- If pH is high and $[HCO_3^-]$ is high, then metabolic alkalosis is the primary disturbance

- If pH is low and $PaCO_2$ is high, then respiratory acidosis is the primary disturbance

- If pH is high and $PaCO_2$ is low, then respiratory alkalosis is the primary disturbance

Step 4 Is compensation appropriate?

- This step is essential for one to understand whether the disturbance is simple (compensation appropriate) or mixed (compensation inappropriate)

- With metabolic acidosis, the $PaCO_2$ (in mmHg) must decrease; conversely, with metabolic alkalosis, the $PaCO_2$ must increase

- Inadequate compensation is equivalent to another primary acid-base disturbance

- It is important to recognize that compensation is never complete; compensatory processes cannot return one's blood pH to what it was before one suffered a primary disturbance; the compensation process itself is not a second acid-base disturbance

TABLE 6–9 (Continued)

Step 5 What is the serum anion gap?

- Calculating the serum anion gap provides insight into the differential diagnosis of metabolic acidosis (anion gap and nonanion gap metabolic acidosis) and can also indicate that metabolic acidosis is present in the patient with an associated metabolic alkalosis

Step 6 If an anion gap is present compare the change in serum anion gap to the change in serum bicarbonate concentration

- If the change in serum anion gap is much larger than the fall in serum bicarbonate concentration, one can infer the presence of both an anion gap metabolic acidosis and metabolic alkalosis

- If the fall in serum bicarbonate concentration is much larger than the increase in the serum anion gap (and the serum anion gap is significantly increased) one can infer the presence of both an anion gap and nonanion gap metabolic acidosis

Step 7 Identify the underlying cause of the disturbance

- This is the whole purpose of analyzing acid-base disorders; one must remember that acid-base disorders are merely laboratory signs of an underlying disease

- The pathologic cause of the acid-base disorder is usually obvious once individual primary disturbances are identified

(continued)

TABLE 6–9 (Continued)

Step 8 Initiate appropriate therapy

- The acid-base disturbance must be directly addressed in several clinical situations. Ultimately, treatment of the underlying cause is most important.

$$[\text{H}^+] = \frac{24 \times \text{PaCO}_2}{[\text{HCO}_3^-]} \qquad (6\text{-}8)$$

The Henderson equation

TABLE 6–10: Conversion of pH to Proton Concentration (nM/L)

6.90 = 125	7.10 = 80	7.30 = 50	7.50 = 32	7.70 = 20
6.92 = 120	7.12 = 76	7.32 = 48	7.52 = 30	7.72 = 19
6.94 = 115	7.14 = 73	7.34 = 46	7.54 = 29	7.74 = 18
6.96 = 110	7.16 = 70	7.36 = 44	7.56 = 28	7.76 = 17
6.98 = 105	7.18 = 66	7.38 = 42	7.58 = 27	7.78 = 17
7.00 = 100	7.20 = 63	7.40 = 40	7.60 = 25	
7.02 = 95	7.22 = 60	7.42 = 37	7.62 = 24	
7.04 = 91	7.24 = 58	7.44 = 35	7.64 = 24	
7.06 = 87	7.26 = 55	7.46 = 33	7.66 = 23	
7.08 = 83	7.28 = 52	7.48 = 33	7.68 = 21	

PATHOPHYSIOLOGY—COMPENSATION AND CONSEQUENCES

TABLE 6–11: Pathophysiologic Mechanisms
Metabolic acidosis is characterized by a primary decrease in $[HCO_3^-]$
Decreased blood pH (acidemia), serum $[HCO_3^-]$ (primary response), and $PaCO_2$ (compensatory response) are the laboratory findings that are the hallmark of simple metabolic acidosis
It is important to keep in mind when evaluating serum electrolytes that not all decreases in serum $[HCO_3^-]$ are the result of metabolic acidosis; metabolic compensation for respiratory alkalosis also reduces serum $[HCO_3^-]$
Mechanisms
• Addition of a strong acid that consumes HCO_3^-
When an organic acid consumes HCO_3^-, the organic anion that is produced is often retained in ECF and serum; in this circumstance, the serum Cl^- concentration does not increase $$HA + NaHCO_3 \rightarrow NaA + H_2CO_3$$
• Loss of HCO_3^- from the body (usually through the GI tract or kidneys)
When HCO_3^- is lost or diluted, an organic anion is not generated

(continued)

TABLE 6–11 (Continued)

Electroneutrality is preserved by reciprocal increases in serum Cl^- concentration; this form of metabolic acidosis is generally referred to as hyperchloremic or nonanion gap metabolic acidosis

$$HCl + NaHCO_3 \rightarrow NaCl + H_2CO_3$$

- Rapid addition of nonbicarbonate-containing solutions to ECF, also called dilutional acidosis

Abbreviations: GI, gastrointestinal; ECF, extracellular fluid

TABLE 6–12: Compensation (Buffering and Respiratory System)

Buffering

The first line of defense against the fall in pH resulting from metabolic acidosis is participation of buffer systems

As a general rule, nonbicarbonate buffers buffer about one-half of an acid load; with more severe acidosis, the participation of nonbicarbonate buffers becomes even more important

Bone contributes importantly to buffering in chronic metabolic acidosis; the attendant Ca^{2+} loss from bone that results in reduced bone density and increased urinary Ca^{2+} excretion are major deleterious consequences of chronic metabolic acidosis

Respiratory system

The $PaCO_2$ declines in the setting of metabolic acidosis; this is a normal, compensatory response

Failure of this normal adaptive response indicates the concomitant presence of respiratory acidosis; this has important clinical significance in that patients who fail to increase ventilation appropriately are 4.2 times more likely to require mechanical ventilation

An excessive decline in $PaCO_2$, producing a normal pH, indicates the presence of concomitant respiratory alkalosis; both situations are considered to be mixed acid-base disturbances

(continued)

TABLE 6–12 (Continued)

The respiratory response to metabolic acidosis is mediated primarily by pH receptors in the central nervous system; peripheral pH receptors probably play a smaller role

The expected $PaCO_2$ can also be calculated using the Winter's formula—$PaCO_2 = 1.5\,[HCO_3^-] + 8 \pm 2$

Even with extremely severe metabolic acidosis the $PaCO_2$ cannot be maintained below $10-15$ mmHg

TABLE 6–13: Compensation (Kidney)

The kidney provides the third and final line of pH defense

This mechanism is relatively slow compared to the immediate effect of buffering and respiratory compensation, which begins within 15–30 min; in contrast, renal compensation requires 3–5 days to become complete

In the presence of normal renal function, acidosis induces increases in NAE by the kidney; the increase in NAE is due primarily to increases in NH_4^+ excretion rather than the minimal changes in phosphate (titratable acid) excretion

Acidosis increases glutamine deamination that generates NH_4^+; NH_4^+ excretion and the ultimate catabolism of α-KG, leads to generation of new HCO_3^-; in fact, there is both transcriptional and translational upregulation of key enzymes involved in glutamine metabolism that are induced by acidosis

Chronic metabolic acidosis also increases renal endothelin-1 that activates the Na^+-H^+ exchanger on the proximal tubule brush border

Acidosis induces both new HCO_3^- generation via the glutamine system and the enhancement of HCO_3^- reabsorption and titratable acid formation; interestingly, decreases in $PaCO_2$ that occur from respiratory compensation, actually limit renal correction of metabolic acidosis

Abbreviations: NAE, net acid excretion; α-KG, alpha-ketoglutarate

TABLE 6–14: Biochemical and Physiological Effects

In the short term, mild degrees of acidemia are often well tolerated; in fact, some physiologic benefit such as increased P_{50} for hemoglobin favoring O_2 delivery to tissues occurs

Cardiovascular effects

If acidosis is severe (pH < 7.10) myocardial contractility and vascular reactivity are depressed; in this setting, hypotension often progresses to profound shock

Acidosis depresses both vascular and myocardial responsiveness to catecholamines; in the case of the vasculature, supraphysiologic concentrations of catecholamines may restore reactivity, but myocardial depression created by acidosis will eventually overcome this effect as pH continues to fall

Metabolic acidosis induces an intracellular acidosis, and this is particularly deleterious to cardiac myocyte function; metabolic acidosis impairs the ability of cardiac myocytes to use energy

On a physiologic level, intracellular acidosis impairs contractile responses to normal and elevated cytosolic Ca^{2+} concentrations

Acidosis induces impairment of actin-myosin cross-bridge cycling

Metabolic acidosis and hypoxia synergistically impair myocardial myocyte metabolism

Respiratory system

With mild degrees of acidosis, it may be difficult to discern an increase in ventilatory effort; more severe metabolic acidosis, pH < 7.20, increases ventilatory effort; this is

TABLE 6–14 (Continued)

readily apparent as respirations become extremely deep and rapid, a clinical sign known as Kussmaul's respiration

Severe metabolic acidosis may result in pulmonary edema

Other organ systems

Bone effects of even mild chronic metabolic acidosis are prominent; this acid-base disturbance leaches Ca^{2+} from bone, resulting in hypercalciuria and bone disease

Normal or increased serum K^+ concentration in the face of decreased total body K^+ stores occurs commonly with metabolic acidosis

- This occurs because acidosis shifts K^+ from the ICF to the ECF, and renal K^+ excretion increases in many states of metabolic acidosis

- Metabolic acidosis is classified as an anion gap (organic) or nonanion gap (hyperchloremic); in general, potassium shifts are more prominent with nonanion gap metabolic acidosis

Abbreviations: ICF, intracellular fluid; ECF, extracellular fluid

USE OF THE SERUM AND URINE ANION GAP IN THE DIFFERENTIAL DIAGNOSIS OF METABOLIC ACIDOSIS

TABLE 6–15: Serum Anion Gap
The SAG is used to determine whether an organic or mineral acidosis is present; this allows the clinician to use simple electrolyte determinations to accurately infer whether an organic anion is present in high concentration
$SAG = [Na^+] - [Cl^-] - [TCO_2]$ we use the TCO_2 as an index of serum bicarbonate
We rather arbitrarily define "unmeasured" as not being in the equation; in other words, UC are those cations that are not Na^+ (e.g., K^+, Mg^{2+}, Ca^{2+}) and UA as anions that are not Cl^- or HCO_3^- (e.g., SO_4^{2-}, $H_2PO_4^-$, HPO_4^{2-}, albumin, and organic anions); the SAG, UA, and UC are expressed in units of mEq/L
Expressed differently $SAG = UA - UC$
For ease of computation, we consider a normal SAG to be about 10 mEq/L, actually it is somewhere between 6 and 10 mEq/L
The SAG is most useful when it is extremely elevated; a major increase in the anion gap (e.g., SAG > 25 mEq/L) always reflects the presence of an organic acidosis
A low SAG is seen in four clinical circumstances: (1) a reduction in the concentration of unmeasured anions (primarily albumin); (2) increased unmeasured cations (hyperkalemia, hypermagnesemia, hypercalcemia, lithium toxicity, or a cationic paraprotein); (3) underestimation of the serum Na^+ concentration (severe hypernatremia); (4) overestimation of the serum Cl^- concentration (bromide intoxication and marked hyperlipidemia)

TABLE 6–15 (Continued)

For each 1 g/dL decrease in serum albumin concentration, the SAG will decrease by 2.5 mEq/L; therefore, in patients with hypoalbuminemia the SAG should be adjusted upward

Abbreviations: SAG, serum anion gap; UC, unmeasured cations; UA, unmeasured anions

FIGURE 6–3: Anion Gap and Nonanion Gap Metabolic Acidosis. If we assume that every proton generated causes a stoichiometric reduction in serum $[HCO_3^-]$ then the addition of organic acid will cause an increase in the SAG, whereas addition of mineral acid (HCl) will not. The SAG is extremely useful in the differential diagnosis of metabolic acidosis. It must be interpreted with some caution. While an organic acidosis should theoretically produce anions in concert with protons, note that the relationship between the increase in SAG and fall in bicarbonate concentration depends primarily on the clearance mechanisms for the anion and the volume of distribution for both bicarbonate and the anion

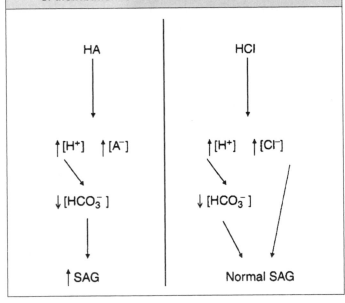

TABLE 6–16: Urine Anion and Osmolar Gap
One cannot routinely measure urinary ammonium concentration; therefore, we must use the same type of reasoning employed for the SAG to develop a method to estimate NH_4^+ concentration based on electrolyte content of urine
Because of electroneutrality we presume—$[Na^+] + [K^+] + UC = [Cl^-] + UA$
When urine pH is < 6, urine does not contain appreciable amounts of bicarbonate; more relevant, the UC is made up mostly of NH_4^+
Therefore, we can define UAG as—$UAG = [Na^+] + [K^+] - [Cl^-]$
It is clear that UAG will be negative when urinary $[NH_4^+]$ is high
UAG is negative because NH_4^+ when excreted in urine is accompanied by Cl^- to maintain charge neutrality
It turns out that low concentrations of urinary NH_4^+ are associated with a positive UAG
UAG is used to differentiate renal (principally tubular acidosis) from nonrenal causes of nonanion gap metabolic acidosis (such as diarrhea)
UAG can be misleading in two clinical circumstances
• The first is when decreased Na^+ delivery compromises distal acid excretion; in order to use the UAG urine Na^+ concentration must be greater than 20 mEq/L; decreased distal Na^+ delivery impairs collecting duct H^+ secretion and UAG cannot be used if Na^+ delivery is decreased

(continued)

TABLE 6–16 (Continued)

• The second occurs when an anion (usually a ketoanion or hippurate) is excreted with Na^+ or K^+; urinary Na^+ and K^+ may be elevated leading to a positive UAG and the impression that the kidney is not responding appropriately; UOG is not affected by excretion of other anions and may need to be used in this situation

$UOG = 2(Na^+ + K^+) + BUN/2.8 + glucose/18$

UOG is not affected by unmeasured urine anions since they are associated with cations (Na^+ or K^+); dividing UOG by 2 will approximate the urinary $[NH_4^+]$; a value less than 40 implies that the kidney is not responding appropriately to metabolic acidosis

Abbreviations: SAG, serum anion gap; UAG, urinary anion gap; UOG, urinary osmolar gap

DIFFERENTIAL DIAGNOSIS OF METABOLIC ACIDOSIS

TABLE 6–17: Differential Diagnosis of Metabolic Acidosis
Examine the serum anion gap
An anion gap metabolic acidosis is characterized by retention of an organic anion (elevated anion gap); in contrast, a hyperchloremic or nonanion gap metabolic acidosis is not associated with retention of an organic anion (normal anion gap)
Anion gap present
Examine blood and urine for ketones to evaluate for ketoacidosis
Lactic acidosis can generally be diagnosed from the clinical presentation; if necessary serum lactate concentration can be measured
After eliminating ketoacidosis and lactic acidosis as potential causes for an anion gap metabolic acidosis one next examines the serum BUN and creatinine concentrations to determine if organic anion accumulation is the result of kidney dysfunction
One must have a high index of suspicion for toxin ingestion; examination of serum osmolar gap and levels of specific toxins can be measured
Anion gap absent
Urinary anion gap can be used to differentiate renal from GI causes of nonanion gap metabolic acidosis if the diagnosis is not obvious based on history and physical examination; the urinary anion gap is equal to the sum of urinary Na^+ and K^+ minus urine Cl^-

(continued)

TABLE 6–17 (Continued)

It will be negative in situations where urinary $[NH_4^+]$ is elevated and the kidney is responding appropriately to metabolic acidosis (nonrenal causes)

In situations where the kidney is responsible for the metabolic acidosis urinary anion gap will be positive; this may occur with either renal tubular acidosis or renal dysfunction; renal dysfunction is identified by elevated serum concentrations of BUN and creatinine

Abbreviations: BUN, blood urea nitrogen; GI, gastrointestinal

CAUSES OF METABOLIC ACIDOSIS

TABLE 6–18: Causes of Increased Anion Gap (Organic) Metabolic Acidosis
Increased acid production
Lactic acidosis
Ketoacidosis
• Diabetic ketoacidosis
• Starvation
• Alcoholic ketoacidosis
Toxic alcohol ingestion
Salicylate overdose
Pyroglutamic acidosis
Other intoxications (e.g., toluene, isoniazid and propylene glycol)
Inborn errors of metabolism
Failure of acid excretion
Acute kidney injury
Chronic kidney disease

TABLE 6–19: Ketoacidosis

There are three forms of anion gap metabolic acidosis that are characterized by ketonemia or ketonuria and these include diabetic ketoacidosis, starvation ketosis, and alcoholic ketoacidosis

In all of these disorders, these is generation and accumulation of short chain fatty ketoacids and hydroxyacids, specifically, acetoacetic acid (ketoacids) and β-hydroxybutyric acid (hydroxyacid)

The urine dipstick uses the Rothera nitroprusside reaction which is most sensitive for acetoacetic acid, has a lower sensitivity for acetone, and does not detect β-hydroxybutyric acid; this can be overcome by either using a dipstick specific for β-hydroxybutyric acid or by adding a few drops of 3% hydrogen peroxide to urine; this will nonenzymatically convert β-hydroxybutyric acid to acetoacetic acid

β-hydroxybutyric acid may make up as much as 90% of ketones in alcoholic ketoacidosis and 75% in diabetic ketoacidosis

FFA from lipolysis can undergo one of three fates:
(1) conversion in liver to triglycerides, CO_2 and H_2O;
(2) conversion into ketoacids or hydroxyacids; and
(3) oxidation to acetyl CoA (blocked by insulin deficiency); in the absence of insulin and presence of enhanced glucagon secretion there is increased lipolysis and FFA delivery to liver, as well as enhanced fatty acyl CoA entry into mitochondria and conversion to ketones

These ketoacids are relatively strong acids that produce acidosis, as well as an increase in anion gap

Abbreviation: FFA, free fatty acids

TABLE 6–20: Diabetic Ketoacidosis
DKA is a common form of anion gap metabolic acidosis
This entity results from a nearly absolute insulin deficiency along with increases in glucagon
The amount of insulin needed for catabolism of short chain fatty acids is significantly less than that necessary for glucose homeostasis; DKA is a common presentation in patients with insulin-dependent diabetes mellitus but is rather unusual in patients with noninsulin-dependent diabetes mellitus
Patients with noninsulin-dependent diabetes mellitus present with marked increases in serum glucose concentrations without ketosis (nonketotic hyperglycemic coma); this entity is also associated with an increase in anion gap, but the chemical nature of accumulated anion(s) is not well characterized
DKA is diagnosed by the combination of anion gap metabolic acidosis, hyperglycemia, and demonstration of increased serum (or urine) ketones; however, presence of serum and urine ketones is not specific for DKA
Elevated ketones may accompany starvation and alcoholic ketoacidosis, where there may be some associated acidosis (see below), as well as isopropyl alcohol intoxication that is characterized by ketosis without significant acidosis
Abbreviation: DKA, diabetic ketoacidosis

TABLE 6–21: Starvation Ketosis

Starvation produces metabolic processes that are similar to those seen with DKA; hepatic ketogenesis is accelerated and tissue ketone metabolism reduced

As carbohydrate availability becomes limited, hepatic ketogenesis is accelerated and tissue ketone metabolism reduced; this produces increases in serum (and urine) concentration of ketoacids and ketones

At first, there is minimal associated acidosis as renal NAE maintains balance; with more prolonged starvation serum $[HCO_3^-]$ often declines; however, it does not generally fall below 18 mEq/L since ketonemia promotes insulin release in patients with a normal pancreas

Abbreviations: DKA, diabetic ketoacidosis; NAE, net acid excretion

TABLE 6–22: Alcoholic Ketoacidosis

AKA is a relatively common form of acidosis seen in inner city hospitals

It results from the combination of alcohol toxicity and starvation; ethanol itself leads to an increase in cytosolic NAD^+, but without glucose (the starvation component), ketogenesis, and decreased ketone usage results

Serum glucose concentration can actually range over a wide spectrum; in some cases it is very low (i.e., < 50 mg/dL), but occasionally it may be moderately high (e.g., 200–300 mg/dL); in the latter circumstance, clinicians may confuse AKA with DKA

Patients with AKA often present with mixed acid-base disorders rather than simple metabolic acidosis

A marked increase in SAG is a hallmark of this disorder

When acidosis is severe, however, the majority of ketoacids circulating in serum may not be detected by the urine dipstick and Acetest assay, which is relatively insensitive to β-hydroxybutyric acid; therefore, a high index of suspicion must be held in the appropriate clinical setting

Abbreviations: AKA, alcoholic ketoacidosis; DKA, diabetic ketoacidosis; SAG, serum anion gap

TABLE 6–23: Lactic Acidosis (L-lactate)

Anaerobic metabolism results in production of lactic acid
Three factors determine lactate concentration: (1) NADH/NAD$^+$ ratio; (2) H$^+$ concentration; and (3) pyruvate concentration; lactate accumulates when there is increased production or decreased utilization; increased production occurs when there is enhanced pyruvate production, decreased utilization occurs most commonly when there is an altered redox state in the cell
NADH is generated during glycolysis and is then reoxidized to NAD$^+$ in mitochondria; if oxidation is impaired NADH accumulates driving the reaction shown in Eq. (6-9) $$H^+ + pyruvate + NADH \rightarrow lactate + NAD^+ \quad (6\text{-}9)$$ The generation of lactate
Aerobic tissues metabolize carbohydrates to pyruvate that then enters an oxidative metabolic pathway (TCA) in mitochondria; this results in regeneration of NAD$^+$ that was consumed in the TCA cycle, as well as in the glycolytic pathway
When tissues perform anaerobic glycolysis NAD$^+$ cannot be regenerated from electron transport; in order to regenerate NAD$^+$, the reaction catalyzed by LDH, must proceed and lactate is generated (Eq. 6-9)
The net effect of glycolysis is to generate lactate from carbohydrates
Normally, lactate (L-isomer) production is closely matched by lactate metabolism to glucose (Cori cycle) or aerobic metabolism to CO$_2$ and H$_2$O, and circulating concentrations are low

TABLE 6–23 (Continued)

Under certain pathologic conditions, there may be a substantial increase in lactate concentration and a concomitant development of metabolic acidosis; these include those with local or systemic decreases in oxygen delivery, impairments in oxidative metabolism, or impaired hepatic clearance; of these local or systemic decreases in O_2 delivery as a result of hypotension are most common

Lactic acidosis is one of the most common forms of anion gap metabolic acidosis; it must be considered as a possible cause of any anion gap metabolic acidosis, particularly if clinical circumstances include hemodynamic compromise, sepsis, tissue ischemia, or hypoxia

Measurement of the serum lactate concentration employs a spectrophotometric assay using the LDH reaction

Medications used to treat HIV may result in lactic acidosis; these include stavudine, zidovudine, and lamivudine

Proton production rate with lactic acidosis (as high as 72 mmol/min) far exceeds its removal rate; for this reason effective treatment always involves correction of the underlying process responsible for lactic acid production

Abbreviations: NAD, nicotinamide adenine dinucleotide; TCA, tricarboxylic acid; LDH, lactate dehydrogenase; HIV, human immunodeficiency virus

TABLE 6–24: Lactic Acidosis (D-lactate)

D-lactic acidosis can be missed since the conventional laboratory assay does not recognize D-lactate

D-lactic acidosis occurs with blind intestinal loops or short bowel syndrome

Excessive amounts of glucose are delivered to the colon where it is metabolized to D-lactate by lactobacilli

Altered mental status is a prominent feature (confusion, memory loss, slurred speech, and ataxia)

The clinician must suspect this diagnosis in the appropriate clinical setting and confirm D-lactic acidosis with alternate measurement methods (e.g., H^+ NMR spectroscopy, HPLC, specific enzymatic method for D-lactate). D-lactate levels are greater than 3 mmol/L

Abbreviation: LDH, lactate dehydrogenase

TABLE 6–25: Chronic Kidney Disease or Acute Kidney Injury

Normally, the kidney is responsible for excretion of approximately 1 mEq/kg/day of H^+ generated from the metabolism of nonvolatile acids and bases and the ingestion of a normal "Western" diet; if the kidney fails to do this, one develops metabolic acidosis

With both acute and chronic kidney injury, there is some retention of anions (including phosphate, sulfate, and some poorly characterized organic anions), and SAG is typically elevated; it is common to find that the increase in SAG is less than the fall in bicarbonate concentration

Renal dysfunction typically gives a mixed anion gap and nonanion gap metabolic acidosis

In renal dysfunction with an anion gap the acid that accumulates is H_2SO_4; this generally does not occur until the glomerular filtration rate is less than 20–30 mL/min

Metabolic acidosis in the setting of acute and chronic kidney injury is generally not severe unless a marked catabolic state occurs, or another acidotic condition (e.g., nonanion gap acidosis from diarrhea) supervenes

Anion gap is generally below 20, serum $[HCO_3^-]$ 12–18 mEq/L, and arterial pH >7.25

Abbreviation: SAG, serum anion gap

TABLE 6–26: Toxic Alcohol Ingestion

Toxic alcohol ingestion should be considered in all patients with an unexplained anion gap metabolic acidosis

Delays in diagnosis and therapy are likely to be accompanied by permanent organ damage and death

These entities are also important to recognize because they often require hemodialysis to remove the offending agent and their metabolites

The most important toxic alcohols include methanol and ethylene glycol; these are often taken as a suicide attempt, but may be inadvertently ingested by children or inebriated adults

While the clinical syndrome ultimately results in very severe metabolic acidosis, it must be stressed that the patient's acid-base status may initially be normal if they present early after ingestion

Because these toxic alcohols are osmotically active, serum osmolar gap (defined as the difference between measured serum osmolarity and calculated serum osmolarity) is used to identify these patients

Serum osmolar gap is generally elevated soon after ingestion because of the presence of the toxic alcohol in serum; if ingestion is remote, it may not be substantially elevated; although useful in suggesting this diagnosis, elevations in serum osmolar gap are neither sensitive nor specific for toxic alcohol ingestion

Ethanol is the most common cause of an elevated serum osmolar gap; therefore, it should be measured and its contribution to the osmolar gap calculated; contribution of ethanol to the osmolar gap is estimated by dividing its concentration in mg/dL by 4.6

TABLE 6–26 (Continued)

Calculated serum osmolarity

$$2[\text{Na}] + \frac{[\text{glucose}]}{18} + \frac{[\text{BUN}]}{2.8} \qquad (6\text{-}10)$$

Serum osmolar gap is equal to measured minus calculated osmolality. Normally the osmolar gap is less than 20 mOsm; [Na^+] is in mEq/L and [glucose] and [BUN] are in mg/dL. This equation can be modified to include additional compounds. The concentration in mg/dL is the numerator and the molecular weight divided by 10 is the denominator. The denominator for some common compounds include: ethanol, 4.6; methanol, 3.2; ethylene glycol, 6.2; acetone, 5.8; and isopropanol, 6.0

TABLE 6–27: Toxic Alcohol Ingestion—Methanol

Methanol intoxication typically presents with abdominal pain, vomiting, headache, and visual disturbances; this latter symptom derives from formic acid toxicity, a methanol metabolite, to the optic nerve; there is generally a lag of 8–30 h from time of ingestion to onset of symptoms

Formic acid is generated via the action of alcohol dehydrogenase

Metabolism is folic acid dependent

Methanol toxicity can be seen with ingestions as small as 30 mL and more than 100 mL is generally fatal unless treated promptly

Seizures, coma or an initial blood pH < 7.0 are associated with high mortality

TABLE 6–28: Toxic Alcohol Ingestion—Ethylene Glycol

Ethylene glycol is a major component of antifreeze; it has a sweet taste that makes it appealing to children, and inebriated adults; it is metabolized by alcohol dehydrogenase to glycolic acid and oxalic acid

Ethylene glycol intoxication presents similarly to that of methanol; both produce CNS disturbances and severe anion gap metabolic acidosis

In contrast to methanol, ethylene glycol does not usually produce retinitis, but may cause both acute and chronic kidney injury

The clinical presentation often consists of three stages: (1) CNS depression that lasts for up to 12 h associated with metabolic acidosis; (2) cardiopulmonary failure; and (3) oliguric acute kidney injury that may be heralded by flank pain

Detection of oxalate crystals in urine is common but may take up to 8 h to appear; calcium oxalate monohydrate crystals may be erroneously interpreted as hippurate crystals by the clinical laboratory

The lethal dose may be as little as 100 mL

Abbreviation: CNS, central nervous system

TABLE 6–29: Toxic Alcohol Ingestion—Treatment

Consideration of either ethylene glycol or methanol ingestion is important because they require very similar and immediate treatment

Neither ethylene glycol nor methanol is particularly toxic in their own right; it is the metabolism of these agents through alcohol dehydrogenase that produces toxic metabolites

Blockade of their metabolism by administration of agents that inhibit alcohol dehydrogenase (ethanol or fomepizole) should be considered early

Moreover, since both parent compounds and metabolites are low molecular weight and have small volumes of distribution, hemodialysis is generally employed; in methanol toxicity hemodialysis is indicated for levels > 50 mg/dL, if acidemia is present, or visual acuity is impaired; with ethylene glycol toxicity hemodialysis is generally employed for levels > 20 mg/dL

Hemodialysis is often required for extended periods of time (approximately 8 h at high blood flows)

It is important to note that if ethanol is used to block metabolism and dialysis is also prescribed, the ethanol dose must be adjusted to compensate for its concomitant removal by dialysis

The loading dose of fomepizole is 15 mg/kg in 100 mL of D5W given over 30 min; maintenance dose is 10 mg/kg every 12 h for 48 h; after 48 h the maintenance dose must be increased to 15 mg/kg every 12 h; since fomepizol induces its own metabolism

(continued)

TABLE 6–29 (Continued)

Fomepizol is cleared by hemodialysis and the interval must be reduced to every 4 h during dialysis; a course of therapy is expensive

If ethanol is used to block alcohol dehydrogenase the level should be maintained between 100 and 200 mg/dL; this requires a loading dose of 0.6 g/kg/h, and a maintenance dose of 0.15 g/kg/h in chronic drinkers and 0.07 g/kg/h in nondrinkers; ethanol is cleared by hemodialysis and the dose must be increased during dialysis

With ethylene glycol intoxication pyridoxine and thiamine promote conversion of glyoxalate to the less toxic metabolites glycine and beta hydroxyketoadipate, respectively

TABLE 6–30: Salicylate Intoxication
Salicylate overdoses are common
Salicylate intoxication may occur as a suicide attempt, but often, especially in the elderly, may result from routine use
Aspirin or methylsalicylate intoxication may lead to serious and mixed acid-base abnormalities
In younger subjects with salicylate intoxication, metabolic acidosis may be simple, whereas in older subjects a mixed acid-base disturbance involving respiratory alkalosis and metabolic acidosis is more likely
Elderly subjects often demonstrate a major discordance between blood concentration and symptoms
CNS toxicity almost always accompanies extremely elevated blood concentration (serum salicylate concentrations > 50 mg/dL)
Salicylates stimulate respiration and produce a component of respiratory alkalosis, especially early in the course of toxicity in adults
Acids responsible for metabolic acidosis and increase in SAG are primarily endogenous acids (e.g., lactate and ketoanions) whose metabolism is affected by toxic amounts of salicylates that uncouple oxidative phosphorylation; salicylic acid contributes to a minor degree
Diagnosis of salicylate toxicity should be considered when a history of aspirin use, nausea, and tinnitus are present; suspicion should also be raised by clinical findings of unexplained respiratory alkalosis, anion gap metabolic acidosis, or noncardiogenic pulmonary edema

(continued)

TABLE 6–30 (Continued)

Advanced age and a delay in diagnosis are associated with significant morbidity and mortality; efforts to remove salicylate include urine alkalinization to a pH of 8.0 with sodium bicarbonate in milder cases

Systemic pH should be carefully monitored and kept below 7.6; hemodialysis is indicated if the salicylate level is > 100 mg/dL, or the patient has altered mental status, depressed GFR, is fluid overloaded or has pulmonary or cerebral edema. Dialysis should also be considered in those that show clinical deterioration despite aggressive supportive measures

Glucose should be administered because CSF glucose concentrations are often low despite normal serum glucose concentration

Acetazolamide should be avoided because it is highly protein bound and may increase free salicylate concentration

Abbreviations: CNS, central nervous system; SAG, serum anion gap; GFR, glomerular filtration rate

TABLE 6–31: Pyroglutamic Acidosis

Mechanism

Pyroglutamic acid is an intermediate compound in the γ-glutamyl cycle that is important in glutathione metabolism and synthesis

Glutathione depletion results in increased formation of γ-glutamyl cysteine that is further metabolized to pyroglutamic acid (also known as 5-oxoproline)

Originally described in patients with a hereditary deficiency of glutathione synthetase

Clinical presentation

Severe anion gap metabolic acidosis, altered mental status, confusion and coma

Most common setting is in the critically ill septic patient given acetaminophen

Critical illness (oxidative stress) and acetaminophen both deplete glutathione

Heterozygous mutations in gluthione synthetase may be a predisposing factor

TABLE 6–32: Other Intoxications

Several other intoxications produce anion gap metabolic acidosis; these include toluene, propylene glycol, strychnine, paraldehyde, iron, isoniazid, papaverine, tetracyclines (outdated), hydrogen sulfide, and carbon monoxide (lactic acidosis)

With citric acid ingestion (present in toilet bowl cleaner) citrate itself causes an increase in SAG; citric acid toxicity is associated with marked hyperkalemia

Toluene is more often associated with a nonanion gap metabolic acidosis; toluene is metabolized to hippurate generating two protons in the process; hippurate is rapidly eliminated from the body by the kidney, and as a consequence the anion does not accumulate leading to a nonanion gap metabolic acidosis; this rather than a distal renal tubular acidosis is the likely mechanism of the normal SAG seen with toluene ingestion

Propylene glycol is associated with both an increased serum anion and osmolar gap. It is used as a solvent for a variety of medications including lorazepam. Each vial of lorazepam contains 830 mg of propylene glycol. When administered at higher than recommended doses (> 0.1 mg/kg/h) it is associated with this syndrome. A critically ill patient should not be given more than 25/mg/kg/day of the solvent

Abbreviation: SAG, serum anion gap

TABLE 6–33: Inborn Errors of Metabolism

Inborn errors of metabolism represent an unusual but important cause of organic acidosis

In some cases (e.g., mitochondrial myopathies, some glycogen storage diseases), lactic acidosis develops without evidence for hypoxia or hypoperfusion

In other conditions (e.g., maple syrup urine disease, methylmalonic aciduria, propionic acidemia, and isovaleric academia), accumulation of other organic acids occurs in concert with metabolic acidosis

Many of these diseases present shortly after birth, some may be first suspected in adulthood

TABLE 6–34: Causes of Hyperchloremic Metabolic Acidosis

Gastrointestinal loss of HCO_3^-

Diarrhea

Gastrointestinal drainage and fistulas

Urinary diversion to bowel

Cl^- containing anion-exchange resins

$CaCl_2$ or $MgCl_2$ ingestion

Renal loss of HCO_3^-

Renal tubular acidosis

Aldosterone deficiency

Pseudohypoaldosteronism

Carbonic anhydrase inhibitors

K^+-sparing diuretics

Miscellaneous causes of hyperchloremic acidosis

Recovery from ketoacidosis

Dilutional acidosis

Addition of HCl

Parenteral alimentation

Sulfur ingestion

TABLE 6–35: Gastrointestinal HCO$_3^-$ Loss-I

Diarrhea

Concentration of HCO_3^- in diarrheal fluid is usually greater than concentration of HCO_3^- in serum

The diagnosis of diarrhea to explain nonanion gap metabolic acidosis may be difficult in the very young or very old who are unable to provide historical details

In general diarrhea must be of large volume (≥ 4 L/day) to generate metabolic acidosis; the normal kidney can produce 200 mmol/day or more of NH_4^+ (enhanced by metabolic acidosis and hypokalemia) generating 200 mmol/day of HCO_3^-; to develop metabolic acidosis one needs either a large volume of diarrhea, decreased renal NH_4^+ production, or excess colonic bacterial organic acid production

When diarrhea causes metabolic acidosis, a significantly negative UAG (i.e., <10 mEq/L) reflecting ample urinary NH_4^+ concentration is present

Patients with all forms of distal RTA have positive UAGs reflecting relatively low urinary [NH_4^+] present in these conditions

Some patients with GI bicarbonate losses will have urine pH > 6.0 due to complete titration of NH_3 to NH_4^+; UAG in these patients will be negative, helping to distinguish those with renal tubular acidosis

Gastrointestinal drainage and fistulas

Intestinal, pancreatic, and biliary secretions have high HCO_3^- and relatively low Cl^- concentrations

Intestine produces approximately 600–700 mL of fluid per day, this may be increased in states of disease

(continued)

TABLE 6–35 (Continued)

Biliary secretions amount to more than 1 L/day; this fluid usually contains $[HCO_3^-]$ as high as 40 mEq/L

Pancreatic secretions are an even greater potential source of bicarbonate loss; volume may exceed 1–2 L/day and contain $[HCO_3^-]$ up to 100 mEq/L

Because of high $[HCO_3^-]$, drainage of these fluids or fistulas can cause significant metabolic acidosis

Abbreviations: UAG, urine anion gap; RTA, renal tubular acidosis

TABLE 6–36: Gastrointestinal HCO_3^- Loss-II
Urinary diversion to bowel
Surgical approaches to bladder and ureteral disease include creation of alternative drainage of urine through in situ bowel and/or conduits produced from excised bowel
Active Cl^-/HCO_3^- exchange by bowel mucosa and intestinal absorption of NH_4^+ can impair renal NAE
Metabolic acidosis is almost certain when a ureterosigmoidostomy is performed
With a ureteroileostomy contact time of urine with intestinal mucosa is short and metabolic acidosis generally does not occur unless there is impaired loop drainage
Cl^- containing anion-exchange resins
Cholestyramine, a resin used to bind bile acids, can also bind HCO_3^-
Cl^-/HCO_3^- exchange across bowel mucosa may be facilitated, and metabolic acidosis may develop; this is most likely in conditions of chronic kidney disease where new HCO_3^- generation is impaired
$CaCl_2$ or $MgCl_2$ ingestion
Ca^{2+} and Mg^{2+} are not absorbed completely in the gastrointestinal tract; unabsorbed Ca^{2+} or Mg^{2+} may bind HCO_3^- in intestinal lumen and facilitate Cl^-/HCO_3^- exchange
Abbreviation: NAE, net acid excretion

TABLE 6–37: Renal HCO_3^- Loss—RTA General Principles

The RTAs are a group of functional disorders that are characterized by an impairment in NAE

We distinguish these conditions from acidosis of renal dysfunction by requiring that impairment in NAE is out of proportion to any reduction in GFR that may be present

In most cases, RTAs occur in patients with a completely normal or near normal GFR

RTAs can be separated based on whether proximal (bicarbonate reabsorption) or distal (bicarbonate regeneration) nephron is primarily involved

It is most simple to divide distal RTAs into those that are associated with hypokalemia and those that are associated with hyperkalemia; the hyperkalemic type is further divided into those due to hypoaldosteronism and those characterized by a generalized defect in Na^+ reabsorption

Distal RTA associated with hypokalemia, also called classic distal RTA was described first, and is referred to as type I RTA; proximal RTA is referred to as type II RTA; there is no type III RTA; finally, distal RTA with hyperkalemia secondary to hypoaldosteronism is referred to as type IV RTA

Abbreviations: RTA, renal tubular acidosis; GFR, glomerular filtration rate; NAE, net acid excretion

TABLE 6–38: Renal HCO_3^- Loss—Proximal RTA
Uncommon in adults
Bicarbonate reabsorption in proximal tubule is impaired, and *plasma threshold* for HCO_3^- is decreased
When plasma $[HCO_3^-]$ exceeds the *plasma threshold* for HCO_3^-, delivery of HCO_3^--rich fluid to distal nephron leads to substantial bicarbonaturia; this is associated with profound urinary K^+ and Na^+ losses
When plasma $[HCO_3^-]$ falls below the *plasma threshold* for HCO_3^-, however, NAE increases and a steady state is achieved
Patients with proximal RTA typically manifest a mild metabolic acidosis with hypokalemia; serum $[HCO_3^-]$ is generally between 14 and 20 mEq/L
If one treats patients with sodium bicarbonate, however, bicarbonaturia recurs, and urinary K^+ losses become severe; patients with proximal RTA require enormous amounts of bicarbonate and K^+ supplementation; some authors discourage treating these patients with alkali
Diagnostically, patients with suspected proximal RTA undergo an infusion with bicarbonate to correct the serum $[HCO_3^-]$; proximal RTA can be diagnosed when fractional HCO_3^- excretion (i.e., fraction of filtered HCO_3^- excreted in urine) exceeds 15%
Proximal RTA may occur as an isolated disturbance of HCO_3^- reabsorption, but more commonly coexists with other defects in proximal nephron function (e.g., reabsorption of glucose, amino acids, phosphate, and uric acid); when generalized proximal tubule function is deranged, the term "Fanconi's syndrome" is used

(continued)

TABLE 6–38 (Continued)
Fanconi's syndrome is complicated by osteomalacia and malnutrition
Proximal RTA may occur as an inherited disorder (Lowe's syndrome, cystinosis, Wilson's disease, hereditary fructose intolerance and tyrosinemia) and present in infancy; alternatively, it may be acquired following exposure to proximal tubular toxins (heavy metals), or in the setting of drug therapy
The most common acquired causes include medications (nucleotide analogues-tenofovir) and multiple myeloma (light chains cause proximal tubular dysfunction)
Abbreviations: RTA, renal tubular acidosis; NAE, net acid excretion

TABLE 6–39: Inherited Forms of Proximal RTA
Generally these disorders present in early childhood
Na$^+$-bicarbonate cotransporter mutations
Loss of function mutation in the basolateral membrane NBCe1
Autosomal recessive-defect in sodium coupled transport
Ocular abnormalities-glaucoma, band keratopathy, and cataracts
Other defects-short stature, hypothyroidism, and cognitive impairment
Carbonic anhydrase II mutations
Autosomal recessive
Presentation also includes osteosclerosis and hepatosplenomegaly
Patients can present with proximal RTA, mixed proximal, and distal RTA or distal RTA
Cystinosis
Autosomal recessive caused by mutations in cystinosin (lysosomal cystine transporter)-endocytic pathway defect
Defect the result of intralysosomal cystine crystal accumulation
Most common inherited form of Fanconi's syndrome
Can present in an infantile and juvenile forms
Diagnosis confirmed by an elevated leukocyte cystine level
Treatment-oral cysteamine every six hours

(continued)

TABLE 6–39 (Continued)
Oculocerebral syndrome of Lowe
X-linked inheritance-endocytic pathway defect
Mutation in phosphoinositol 4,5-bisphosphate phosphatase
Also involves the eye and nervous system
Renal involvement includes Fanconi's syndrome and progressive renal failure
Occasional hypercalciuria
Dent's disease
X-linked inheritance-endocytic pathway defect
Inactivating mutations of the chloride channel CLC-5 which is coexpressed with vacuolar ATPase in endosomes
Plays a key role in endosomal acidification
Hypercalciuria is common while metabolic acidosis is rare
Abbreviations: RTA, renal tubular acidosis; NBC, sodium bicarbonate cotransporter

TABLE 6–40: Renal HCO_3^- Loss—Distal RTA

Although classic type I distal RTA was initially characterized by an impairment in urinary acidification, all distal RTAs result in an impairment in NAE; this is largely due to reduced urinary NH_4^+ excretion

Type I distal RTA may be associated with either hypokalemia or hyperkalemia

RTA associated with hyperkalemia is the most common form, generally resulting from hypoaldosteronism

All distal RTAs are characterized by a positive UAG in the setting of acidosis, reflecting inadequate NH_4^+ excretion

Abbreviations: RTA, renal tubular acidosis; NAE, net acid excretion; UAG, urine anion gap

TABLE 6–41: Renal HCO_3^- Loss—Distal RTA Hypokalemic

Hypokalemic type I distal RTA is best considered a disorder of collecting duct capacity for effective proton secretion such that patients cannot achieve the necessary NAE to maintain acid-base balance

Patients with hypokalemic type I distal RTA usually present with hyperchloremic metabolic acidosis but are unable to acidify their urine (below pH 5.5) despite systemic acidosis

Two mechanisms were suggested for impaired acidification by distal nephron in hypokalemic distal RTA; back leak of acid through a "leaky" epithelium and proton pump failure (i.e., the H^+ ATPase cannot pump sufficient amounts of H^+)

Hypokalemic type I distal RTA may be inherited or may be associated with other acquired disturbances

Some of the same conditions that can cause hypokalemic distal RTA (e.g., urinary obstruction, autoimmune disorders) can also cause hyperkalemic distal RTA due to a defect in Na^+ reabsorption, suggesting that the mechanistic analysis discussed above might be somewhat artificial

In its primary form, hypokalemic type I distal RTA is unusual, and generally diagnosed in young children; afflicted children typically present with severe metabolic acidosis, growth retardation, nephrocalcinosis, and nephrolithiasis

Hypokalemia, which is usually present, may actually be caused by associated Na^+ depletion and stimulation of the renin-angiotensin-aldosterone axis

TABLE 6–41 (Continued)

Renal K^+ losses decrease considerably when appropriate therapy with sodium bicarbonate is instituted; this is completely different from patients with proximal RTA where urinary K^+ losses increase during therapy because of bicarbonaturia

Proton pump failure can be documented, if necessary, by measuring urinary PCO_2; in an alkaline urine (pH > 7.4) the major H^+ acceptor is HCO_3^-; a HCO_3^- load (0.5–2.0 mmol/kg oral or 2.75% $NaHCO_3$ 4 ml/kg/hr intravenously) may be required to achieve this; patients with normal H^+ secretion will have a urinary PCO_2 > 70 mmHg (or 30 mmHg > blood PCO_2), while those with secretory defects will have a urinary PCO_2 <50 mmHg

Abbreviations: RTA, renal tubular acidosis; NAE, net acid excretion

TABLE 6–42: Inherited Forms of Distal RTA

Secondary to mutations in proteins expressed in the alpha intercalated cell

All present with metabolic acidosis, hypokalemia, and growth retardation

AE1 (SLC4A1) mutations

Functions as a basolateral chloride bicarbonate exchanger

Autosomal dominant, rarely autosomal recessive

Presentation also includes nephrocalcinosis and bilateral sensorineural hearing loss

H^+ ATPase mutations

Mutations described in ATPase V1 subunit B, isoform 1 and V0 subunit A, isoform 4

Autosomal recessive

Presentation also includes nephrocalcinosis, and can include hearing loss

Carbonic anhydrase II mutations

Autosomal recessive

Presentation also includes osteosclerosis and hepatosplenomegaly

Patients can present with proximal RTA, mixed proximal, and distal RTA or distal RTA

Abbreviations: RTA, renal tubular acidosis; AE1, anion exchange protein 1; ATP, adenosine triphosphate

TABLE 6–43: Renal HCO_3^- Loss—Distal RTA Hyperkalemic

Hyperkalemic distal RTAs can develop from: (1) a defect in Na^+ reabsorption where a favorable transepithelial voltage cannot be generated and/or maintained, and (2) hypoaldosteronism

Distal RTA—defect in Na^+ reabsorption

Hyperkalemic distal RTA from decreased Na^+ reabsorption is more common than either classic hypokalemic type I distal RTA or proximal RTA

Urinary obstruction is the most common cause; other causes include cyclosporine nephrotoxicity, renal allograft rejection, sickle cell nephropathy, and many autoimmune disorders such as lupus nephritis and Sjögren's syndrome

In contrast to hypoaldosteronism, urinary acidification is impaired

Hyperkalemia plays a less significant role in the pathogenesis of impaired NH_4^+ excretion, which is more closely tied to impaired distal nephron function

Distal RTA—hypoaldosteronism

Distal RTA from hypoaldosteronism results from either selective aldosterone deficiency or complete adrenal insufficiency

The most common form of RTA is a condition called hyporeninemic hypoaldosteronism (type IV RTA) that is most often seen in patients afflicted with diabetic nephropathy

Urinary acidification assessed by urine pH is normal but NAE is low

(continued)

TABLE 6–43 (Continued)

The defect in NAE in some of these patients can be explained by impaired NH_4^+ synthesis in proximal nephron resulting directly from hyperkalemia

Hyperkalemia also interferes with NH_4^+ recycling in the thick ascending limb of Henle where it competes with NH_4^+ on the K^+ site of the Na^+-K^+-$2Cl^-$ cotransporter

Other patients with hyporeninemic hypoaldosteronism have a more complex pathophysiology

Abbreviations: RTA, renal tubular acidosis; NAE, net acid excretion

TABLE 6–44: Etiologies of Aldosterone Deficiency
Addison's disease
21 hydroxylase deficiency
Bilateral adrenalectomy
Adrenal gland hemorrhage
Hyporeninemic hypoaldosteronism (type IV RTA)
Medications
Spironolactone
Heparin
NSAIDs
Angiotensin-converting enzyme inhibitors and receptor blockers
Pseudohypoaldosteronism (types I and II)
Abbreviations: RTA; renal tubular acidosis; NSAIDs, nonsteroidal anti-inflammatory drugs

TABLE 6–45: Pseudohypoaldosteronism

Type I

Autosomal recessive and dominant forms

Recessive—loss of function of ENaC

- Salt wasting, hypotension, hyperkalemia, neonatal presentation

Dominant—inactivating mutations in the mineralocorticoid receptor

- Salt wasting and hyperkalemia that improves with age

Type II—Gordon's syndrome

Autosomal dominant inheritance

Hyperkalemia, hypertension, metabolic acidosis

Result of WNK1 and WNK4 mutations-serine/threonine kinases

WNK4—loss of function mutation results in increased activity of NCC in the apical membrane of the DCT

WNK1—gain of function mutation results in increased inhibition of WNK4 and increased activity of NCC and ENaC

Both mutations result in increased endocytosis of ROMK and hyperkalemia

Abbreviations: ENaC, epithelial Na^+ channel; WNK, with no lysine; NCC, sodium chloride cotransporter; DCT, distal convoluted tubule

TABLE 6–46: Renal HCO_3^- Loss—Other Causes

CA inhibitors

CA inhibitors (e.g., acetazolamide) inhibit both proximal tubular luminal brush border (type IV isoform) and cellular carbonic anhydrase (type II isoform)

Disruption of CA results in impaired HCO_3^- reabsorption similar to proximal RTA

Topiramate is an antiseizure medication that causes a mild-to-moderate proximal RTA through this mechanism

The antiepileptic drug zonisamide also inhibits carbonic anhydrase

K^+ sparing diuretics

Aldosterone antagonists (e.g., spironolactone and eplerenone) or Na^+ channel blockers (e.g., amiloride and triamterene) may also produce hyperchloremic acidosis in concert with hyperkalemia

Trimethoprim and pentamidine may also function as Na^+ channel blockers and cause hyperkalemia and hyperchloremic metabolic acidosis; this is most often seen in HIV-infected patients

Abbreviations: CA, carbonic anhydrase; RTA, renal tubular acidosis; HIV, human immunodeficiency virus

TABLE 6–47: Miscellaneous Causes

Recovery from ketoacidosis

Patients with DKA generally present with a "pure" anion gap metabolic acidosis; the increase in anion gap roughly parallels the fall in bicarbonate concentration; however, during therapy, renal perfusion is often improved, and substantial loss of ketoanions in urine may result

Many patients afflicted with DKA may eliminate ketoanion faster than they correct their acidosis, leaving them with a nonanion gap or hyperchloremic metabolic acidosis; rarely, this phenomenon may occur in patients who drink enough fluid to maintain GFR close to normal as they develop DKA

Dilutional acidosis

The rapid, massive expansion of ECF volume with fluids that do not contain HCO_3^- (e.g., 0.9% saline) can dilute plasma $[HCO_3^-]$ and cause a mild, nonanion gap metabolic acidosis

This is occasionally seen with trauma resuscitation or during treatment of right ventricular myocardial infarction

Addition of hydrochloric acid

Therapy with HCl or one of its congeners (e.g., ammonium chloride or lysine chloride) will rapidly consume HCO_3^-, and thus, cause hyperchloremic metabolic acidosis

Parenteral alimentation

Amino acid infusions may produce a hyperchloremic metabolic acidosis in a manner similar to addition of HCl

TABLE 6–47 (Continued)

This occurs commonly if alkali-generating compounds (e.g., acetate or lactate) are not administered concomitantly with amino acids; replacement of the Cl^- salt of these amino acids with an acetate salt avoids this problem

Metabolism of sulfur containing amino acids obligates excretion of acid since neutrally charged sulfur is excreted as sulfate; in general, 1 g of amino acid mixture requires 1 mEq of acid to be excreted; acetate content of parenteral alimentation should match the amino acid content on a mEq/g basis

Abbreviations: DKA, diabetic ketoacidosis; GFR, glomerular filtration rate; ECF, extracellular fluid

TREATMENT OF METABOLIC ACIDOSIS

TABLE 6–48: Treatment
The fundamental principles of acid-base therapy are that a *diagnosis must be made* and *treatment of the underlying disease state* initiated; that said, some direct therapy of metabolic acidosis is sometimes indicated
Metabolic acidosis—nonanion gap (hyperchloremic)
With most hyperchloremic metabolic acidoses gradual correction of acidosis is effective and beneficial
Oral bicarbonate or an anion that can be metabolized to bicarbonate is generally preferred
• One gram of sodium bicarbonate is equivalent to 12 mEq of HCO_3^-; in order to administer 1 mEq/kg/day, doses will generally exceed 5 g/day in adults
• Commercially available sodium or mixed sodium and potassium citrate solutions (e.g., Shohl's solution and Bicitra 1mEq/ml or Polycitra syrup 2 mEq/ml) contain 1–2 mEq of HCO_3^- equivalent per mL; citrate solutions may be better tolerated than sodium bicarbonate tablets or powder (baking soda); however, citrate can increase GI absorption of aluminum and should not be administered along with aluminum-based phosphate binders
Metabolic acidosis—increased anion gap
The acute treatment of metabolic acidosis associated with an increased anion gap with IV sodium bicarbonate is controversial; there are two controlled trials showing it as ineffective

TABLE 6–48 (Continued)

Based primarily on experimental models, it appears that bicarbonate therapy may be deleterious in this setting, especially if acidosis is associated with impaired tissue perfusion; the so-called "paradoxical" intracellular acidosis that results when bicarbonate is infused during metabolic acidosis probably accounts for a portion of these deleterious effects

Hypertonic sodium bicarbonate therapy in the form of 50 mL ampules of 1 M $NaHCO_3$ may promote hypertonicity the hypertonic state itself may impair cardiac function, especially in patients undergoing resuscitation for cardiac arrest

Based on these data, we do not support therapy with IV sodium bicarbonate for acute anion gap metabolic acidosis in the emergency situation

Abbreviation: IV, intravenous

FIGURE 6–4: Paradoxical Intracellular Acidosis. This is a direct consequence of the greater permeability of cell membranes to CO_2 than HCO_3^-. Addition of HCO_3^- to blood (or an organism) produces CO_2. When metabolic acidosis is present, more CO_2 is produced for a given dose of sodium bicarbonate than if there were no acidosis. Recent studies performed in a closed, human blood model demonstrate that production of CO_2 from administered HCO_3^- is directly dependent on initial pH. When ventilation is normal, the lungs rapidly eliminate this extra CO_2; however, when pulmonary ventilation, or more commonly tissue ventilation, is impaired (by poor tissue perfusion) CO_2 generated by infused HCO_3^- may diffuse into cells (Far more rapidly than the original HCO_3^- molecule) and paradoxically decrease intracellular pH. Experimentally, administration of sodium bicarbonate in models of metabolic acidosis is associated with a fall in intracellular pH in several organs including heart

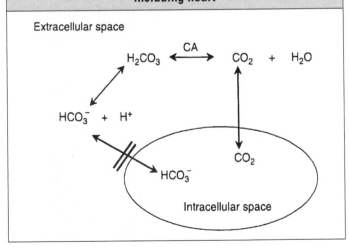

7
Metabolic Alkalosis

INTRODUCTION

Metabolic alkalosis is an acid-base disorder that occurs as the result of a process that increases pH (alkalemia) due to a primary increase in serum $[HCO_3^-]$

TABLE 7–1: Pathophysiology of Metabolic Alkalosis
Net H^+ loss from the ECF
A loss of protons from the body occurs primarily through either the kidneys or the GI tract
When H^+ losses exceed the daily H^+ load produced by metabolism and diet, a net negative H^+ balance results; because the H^+ loss results in generation of a HCO_3^-, increases in serum $[HCO_3^-]$ result
GI proton loss generally occurs in stomach; in this setting, H^+ secretion by the luminal gastric parietal cell H^+ ATPase leaves a HCO_3^- to be reclaimed at the basolateral surface
In kidney, there is also coupling between net acid excretion and bicarbonate generation
Net bicarbonate or bicarbonate precursor addition to the ECF
HCO_3^- administration or addition of substances that generate HCO_3^- (e.g., lactate, citrate) at a rate greater than that of metabolic H^+ production leads to an increase in ECF $[HCO_3^-]$

(continued)

TABLE 7–1 (Continued)

With normal kidney function ECF [HCO_3^-] will not increase significantly; this occurs because as serum [HCO_3^-] exceeds the PT for HCO_3^- reabsorption, the kidney excretes the excess HCO_3^-; as a result serum bicarbonate will not rise unless there is a change in renal bicarbonate handling (maintenance factor)

Loss of fluid from the body that contains Cl^- in greater concentration and bicarbonate in lower concentration than serum-contraction alkalosis

If this type of fluid is lost ECF volume must contract and if contraction is substantial enough, a measurable increase in serum [HCO_3^-] develops

Bicarbonate is now distributed in a smaller volume resulting in an absolute increase in ECF [HCO_3^-]

Abbreviations: ECF, extracellular fluid; GI, gastrointestinal; PT, plasma threshold

TABLE 7–2: Compensation for Metabolic Alkalosis

The normal kidney has a powerful protective mechanism against the development of significant increases in ECF $[HCO_3^-]$, namely the PT for $[HCO_3^-]$ above which proximal reabsorption fails and HCO_3^- losses in urine begin; in almost all cases of metabolic alkalosis the kidney must participate in the pathophysiology; exceptions occur when renal function is dramatically impaired (e.g., chronic kidney disease or acute kidney injury) and/or when ongoing alkali load truly overwhelms renal capacity for bicarbonate elimination (rare)

Pathophysiology involves initiation factors and maintenance factors (those that prevent renal excretion of excess bicarbonate); metabolic alkalosis occurs when the kidney's ability to raise the PT for $[HCO_3^-]$ is impaired (maintenance factor)

Mechanisms

Acute

The first line of pH defense is buffering

When HCO_3^- is added to ECF, protons react with some of this HCO_3^- to produce CO_2 that is normally exhaled by the lungs; through this chemical reaction, the increase in serum and ECF $[HCO_3^-]$ is attenuated; the ICF contributes the majority of H^+ used in this process

Respiratory compensation also occurs; respiratory compensation to metabolic alkalosis follows the same principles as respiratory compensation to metabolic acidosis; the direction of the $PaCO_2$ change is different (i.e., hypercapnia due to hypoventilation rather than hypocapnia due to hyperventilation) and constraints regarding oxygenation limit the magnitude of this hypoventilatory response

(continued)

TABLE 7–2 (Continued)
With metabolic alkalosis, the $PaCO_2$ should increase 0.6–1.0 times the increase in serum $[HCO_3^-]$; absence of compensation constitutes coexistence of a secondary respiratory disturbance
Chronic
Chronic compensation is mediated via the kidney
In a manner analogous to tubular reabsorption of glucose, we can consider the maximal amount of tubular bicarbonate reabsorption (T_{max}) as the PT above which bicarbonaturia occurs; once PT is exceeded, urinary bicarbonate excretion is proportional to GFR
The kidney can excrete large amounts of bicarbonate; for example, if GFR is 100 mL/min and bicarbonate concentration is 10 mEq/L above PT, bicarbonate will be lost in urine initially at a rate of 1 mEq/min
The response by the kidney to excrete excessive HCO_3^- will correct metabolic alkalosis unless there is a maintenance factor that prevents this
Abbreviations: ECF, extracellular fluid; PT, plasma threshold; GFR, glomerular filtration rate

MAINTENANCE OF METABOLIC ALKALOSIS

FIGURE 7–1: Maintenance of Metabolic Alkalosis. A number of factors increase the apparent T_{max} for HCO_3^-. As a result, they increase net HCO_3^- reabsorption by the kidney

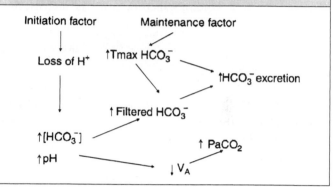

TABLE 7–3: Maintenance Factors

Arterial blood volume decrease

Volume depletion either absolute (e.g., salt losses through vomiting or bleeding) or effective (e.g., congestive heart failure, nephrotic syndrome, hepatic cirrhosis) increase the T_{max} and PT for HCO_3^- reabsorption

Proximal (increased proximal tubule reabsorption of Na^+ and water) and distal (mineralocorticoid effect) mechanisms play a role in the process

Catecholamines and AII stimulate the Na^+-H^+ exchanger isoform in the luminal membrane of proximal tubule (NHE3); proton excretion into urine generates bicarbonate that is transported across the basolateral membrane into blood

Mineralocorticoids act distally to directly stimulate the H^+ ATPase, and indirectly raise the driving force for proton excretion by increasing lumen electronegativity (through stimulation of the epithelial Na^+ channel)

Cl^- depletion

Na^+ and Cl^- losses result in ECF volume depletion

Cl^- depletion also has effects that are independent of ECF volume

Aldosterone

Mineralocorticoids increase distal Na^+ reabsorption which, in turn, increases renal HCO_3^- generation and effectively raises PT and T_{max} for HCO_3^-; these effects can occur in the absence of decreases in effective arterial blood volume

TABLE 7–3 (Continued)

Aldosterone's predominant effect is in distal nephron; shown in Figure 7–2 is a model of two of the three major cell types in collecting duct, the principal cell and alpha-intercalated cell

K^+ depletion

K^+ depletion increases the apparent T_{max} and PT for HCO_3^- and, thus, acts as a maintenance factor for metabolic alkalosis

K^+ depletion may promote a relative intracellular acidosis and this relative intracellular acidosis makes renal H^+ excretion more favorable; however, there is evidence against this concept

- Investigators failed to detect a decrease in renal intracellular pH during experimental K^+ depletion with ^{31}P NMR spectroscopy

- In human studies, metabolic alkalosis can be corrected almost completely without correction of K^+ depletion

K^+ depletion results in cellular K^+ depletion in proximal tubule; this hyperpolarizes the basolateral membrane and increases the driving force for bicarbonate exit via the Na^+-$3HCO_3^-$ cotransporter

K^+ depletion upregulates H^+-K^+ ATPase in the collecting duct intercalated cell; it is likely that this upregulation results in increased H^+ secretion and HCO_3^- generation

(continued)

TABLE 7–3 (Continued)
Hypercapnia
The apparent T_{max} and PT for HCO_3^- are raised by increases in $PaCO_2$; this is related to decreases in intracellular pH that occur during acute and chronic hypercapnia
Although increases in $PaCO_2$ are part of the normal respiratory compensation, they impair the kidney's ability to return serum bicarbonate concentration to normal
Abbreviations: PT, plasma threshold; AII, angiotensin II; ATP, adenosine triphosphate; ECF, extracellular fluid

FIGURE 7–2: Cell Types of the Collecting Duct. The principal cell is responsible for Na$^+$ reabsorption and K$^+$ secretion. The alpha-intercalated cell mediates acid secretion and, therefore, bicarbonate reabsorption and generation. K$^+$ secretion is passive and dependent strictly on the electro-chemical gradient. K$^+$ secretion can be increased by raising intracellular K$^+$, lowering luminal K$^+$, or making the lumen more electronegative

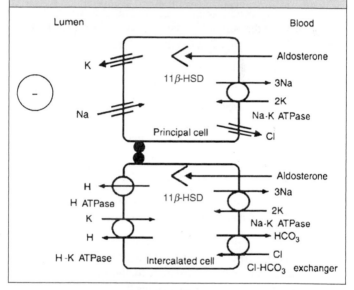

TABLE 7–4: Mechanisms of Aldosterone Action

Effects on H^+ secretion in the distal nephron

Aldosterone directly stimulates H^+ ATPase present in the luminal membrane of the intercalated cell

It also acts indirectly by increasing lumen electronegativity (through Na^+ reabsorption)

Effects on K^+ secretion in the distal nephron

Stimulation of the Na^+-K^+ ATPase increases intracellular K^+ resulting in an increase in the driving force for K^+ secretion

In the long-term aldosterone increases the expression of the Na^+-K^+ ATPase in the principal cell

Aldosterone increases distal Na^+ reabsorption by causing the insertion of Na^+ channels, as well as synthesis of new Na^+ channels; the increase in luminal electronegativity increases the driving force for K^+ secretion

Cellular actions of aldosterone

Aldosterone binds to its receptor in the cytoplasm; this complex translocates to the nucleus and stimulates gene transcription

The specificity of aldosterone's effect does not occur at the level of the receptor; it was found that glucocorticoids have similar affinity to that of aldosterone for the mineralocorticoid receptor and circulate at many times the concentration

Collecting duct cells possess the enzyme type II 11β-HSD that degrades active cortisol to inactive cortisone; ensuring that any cortisol entering the collecting duct cell will be inactivated

If type II 11β-HSD is congenitally absent (apparent mineralocorticoid excess), inhibited (licorice, carbenoxolone and bioflavinoids), or overwhelmed (Cushing's syndrome) glucocorticoids can exert a mineralocorticoid-like effect in collecting duct

Abbreviations: HSD, hydroxysteroid dehydrogenase; ATP, adenosine triphosphate

CLINICAL FEATURES

TABLE 7–5: Clinical Features of Metabolic Alkalosis
Signs and symptoms
Signs and symptoms are nonspecific
Patients who present with muscle cramps, weakness, arrhythmias, or seizures, especially in the setting of diuretic use and vomiting, should prompt consideration of metabolic alkalosis
Most signs and symptoms are due to decreases in ionized Ca^{2+} that occur as the increased pH causes plasma proteins to bind Ca^{2+} more avidly
At a pH above 7.6 malignant ventricular arrhythmias and seizures may be seen
Humans tolerate alkalosis less well than acidosis
Compensation
Examination of arterial blood gases will demonstrate an increased pH, increased $[HCO_3^-]$, and increased $PaCO_2$ with the increase in $PaCO_2$ being between 0.6 and 1 times the increase in $[HCO_3^-]$
Associated electrolyte abnormalities
Serum electrolytes reveal increased serum bicarbonate concentration or more precisely elevated total CO_2 content (TCO_2), which is the sum of the serum $[HCO_3^-]$ and dissolved CO_2, decreased Cl^- concentration and, typically, decreased K^+ concentration

(continued)

TABLE 7–5 (Continued)
Hypokalemia occurs predominantly from enhanced renal K^+ losses
• Increased renal K^+ excretion results from maintenance factors involved in the pathogenesis of metabolic alkalosis
• Elevated mineralocorticoid concentration (or substances with mineralocorticoid-like activity) are almost always involved as a maintenance factor
• Severe metabolic alkalosis may be associated with an increased SAG (increases up to 10–12 mEq/L)
• The majority of the increase is due to increased electronegativity of albumin with elevated pH
• Small increases in lactate concentration resulting from enhanced glycolysis secondary to disinhibition of phosphofructokinase also contribute
Abbreviation: SAG, serum anion gap

DIFFERENTIAL DIAGNOSIS

FIGURE 7–3: Approach to the Patient with Metabolic Alkalosis. The first step in evaluation of the patient with metabolic alkalosis is to subdivide them into those that have ECF Cl^- depletion as a maintenance factor (Cl^- responsive) from those that do not (Cl^- resistant). This is accomplished by measuring urinary Cl^-. At first glance this might be surprising since urinary Na^+ concentration and fractional excretion of Na^+ are examined most commonly as indicators of volume depletion. These may be misleading in metabolic alkalosis, however, especially if the kidney is excreting bicarbonate that will obligate increased Na^+ excretion. In general, Cl^--responsive metabolic alkalosis corrects when volume expansion or improvement of hemodynamics occurs. In contrast, Cl^--resistant metabolic alkalosis does not correct with these maneuvers. Patients with Cl^--responsive metabolic alkalosis typically have urine Cl^- concentrations less than 20 mEq/L, whereas patients with Cl^--resistant metabolic alkalosis have urine Cl^-concentrations exceeding 20 mEq/L

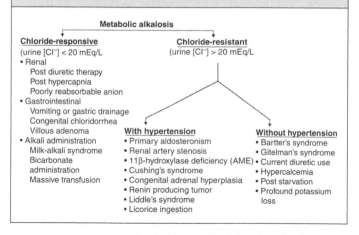

Metabolic alkalosis

Chloride-responsive
(urine [Cl^-] < 20 mEq/L
• Renal
  Post diuretic therapy
  Post hypercapnia
  Poorly reabsorbable anion
• Gastrointestinal
  Vomiting or gastric drainage
  Congenital chloridorrhea
  Villous adenoma
• Alkali administration
  Milk-alkali syndrome
  Bicarbonate administration
  Massive transfusion

Chloride-resistant
(urine [Cl^-] > 20 mEq/L

With hypertension
• Primary aldosteronism
• Renal artery stenosis
• 11β-hydroxylase deficiency (AME)
• Cushing's syndrome
• Congenital adrenal hyperplasia
• Renin producing tumor
• Liddle's syndrome
• Licorice ingestion

Without hypertension
• Bartter's syndrome
• Gitelman's syndrome
• Current diuretic use
• Hypercalcemia
• Post starvation
• Profound potassium loss

TABLE 7–6: Causes of Cl⁻-Responsive Metabolic Alkalosis
Gastrointestinal causes
Vomiting or gastric drainage
Colonic villous adenoma
Cl⁻ diarrhea
Renal causes
Diuretic therapy
Posthypercapnia
Poorly reabsorbable anions
Exogenous alkali administration or ingestion
Bicarbonate administration
Milk-alkali syndrome
Transfusion of blood products (sodium citrate)

TABLE 7–7: Causes of Cl⁻-Resistant Metabolic Alkalosis

With hypertension

Primary aldosteronism

Renal artery stenosis

Renin-producing tumor

Cushing's syndrome

Licorice or chewing tobacco, carbenoxolone

Apparent mineralocorticoid excess

Congenital adrenal hyperplasia

Liddle's syndrome

Without hypertension

Bartter syndrome

Gitelman's syndrome

Current diuretic use

Profound K^+ depletion

Hypercalcemia (nonhyperparathyroid etiology)

Poststarvation (refeeding alkalosis)

CL⁻-RESPONSIVE AND CL⁻-RESISTANT CAUSES OF METABOLIC ALKALOSIS

TABLE 7–8: GI and Renal Causes of Cl⁻-Responsive Metabolic Alkalosis
Vomiting and gastric drainage
Patients with persistent vomiting or nasogastric suctioning may lose up to 2 L/day of fluid containing a proton concentration of 100 mmol/L
Gastric parietal cells excrete up to 200 mmol of HCO_3^- per day; this constitutes a significant initiation factor; however, it is the Na^+, Cl^-, and K^+ losses that allow metabolic alkalosis to be maintained
K^+ losses are more significant in urine than in vomitus that generally contains only about 10 mEq/L of K^+
Colonic villous adenoma
Rarely a colonic villous adenoma has significant secretory potential
The adenoma produces profound diarrhea that contains excessive amounts of protein, Na^+, K^+, Cl^- and relatively low HCO_3^- concentration; this leads to metabolic alkalosis—in contrast to the typical metabolic acidosis that more commonly complicates diarrheal states
Congenital chloridorrhea
Congenital chloridorrhea is a rare congenital syndrome arising from a defect in small and large bowel Cl^- absorption causing chronic diarrhea with a fluid that is rich in Cl^- leading to metabolic alkalosis
Results from a mutation in the DRA gene; DRA functions as a Cl^--bicarbonate and Cl^--sulfate exchanger and is expressed in the apical membrane of colonic epithelium

TABLE 7–8 (Continued)
Diuretic therapy
Loop diuretics that exert their effects in the TALH (e.g., furosemide, bumetanide) and thiazide diuretics that act in distal tubule (e.g., hydrochlorothiazide, and metolazone) may facilitate volume depletion, as well as directly stimulate renin secretion (loop diuretics); these diuretics can, thus, provide both initiation and maintenance factors and produce metabolic alkalosis
If the diuretic is still active urinary Cl^- concentration is typically elevated; if the diuretic is no longer active (typically 24–48 h after a dose) urinary Cl^- concentration is low
Metabolic alkalosis associated with hypokalemia is a common complication of diuretic use, and should suggest the possibility of diuretic abuse; diuretics are commonly abused in patients with anorexia nervosa
Abbreviations: GI, gastrointestinal; DRA, downregulated in adenoma; TALH, thick limb of Henle

TABLE 7–9: Miscellaneous Causes of Cl⁻-Responsive Metabolic Alkalosis-I

Posthypercapnia

The kidney responds to chronic elevations in $PaCO_2$ by raising the plasma HCO_3^- concentration; if hypercapnia is subsequently corrected rapidly, as occurs with intubation and mechanical ventilation, the elevated serum HCO_3^- concentration will persist for at least several hours until renal correction is complete

Sufficient Cl^- must be present to allow for this renal correction, and many patients with diseases leading to hypercapnia are also treated with diuretics that may cause Cl^- depletion

Poorly reabsorbable anions

Large doses of some lactam antibiotics, such as penicillin and carbenicillin, may result in hypokalemic metabolic alkalosis

The initiation and maintenance factor is the delivery of large quantities of poorly reabsorbable anions to the distal nephron with attendant increases in H^+ and K^+ excretion

Cystic fibrosis

Metabolic alkalosis may develop in children with cystic fibrosis due to Cl^- losses in sweat that has a low $[HCO_3^-]$

The maintenance factor is resultant volume depletion caused by these losses

TABLE 7–9 (Continued)

Alkali administration

Patients with chronic kidney disease whose ability to excrete a HCO_3^- load is decreased may develop sustained metabolic alkalosis following alkali administration

Baking soda is the richest source of exogenous alkali containing 60 mEq of bicarbonate per teaspoon; many patients ingest baking soda as a "home remedy" to treat dyspepsia and various GI problems

Substances whose metabolism yields HCO_3^- (citrate or acetate) may be an alkali source

Abbreviation: GI, gastrointestinal

TABLE 7–10: Miscellaneous Causes of Cl⁻-Responsive Metabolic Alkalosis–II

Milk-alkali syndrome

The milk-alkali syndrome is classically noted in patients with GI upset who consume large amounts of antacids containing Ca^{2+} and absorbable alkali; calcium carbonate or Tums is most often ingested for this purpose

Volume depletion (or at least the lack of ECF volume expansion) along with hypercalcemia-mediated suppression of parathyroid hormone secretion contributes to maintenance of metabolic alkalosis

Hypercalcemia decreases renal blood flow and glomerular filtration, reducing the filtered load of bicarbonate and further impairing renal correction of metabolic alkalosis

Nephrocalcinosis may develop with chronic antacid ingestion, a pathologic factor that decreases GFR further, and more profoundly reduces the kidney's ability to excrete an alkali load

Transfusion of blood products

Infusion of more than 10 units of blood containing the anticoagulant citrate can produce a moderate metabolic alkalosis analogous to alkali administration

In many cases, some degree of GFR reduction may contribute to the maintenance of metabolic alkalosis

Through an identical mechanism, patients given parenteral hyperalimentation with excessive amounts of acetate or lactate may also develop metabolic alkalosis

Abbreviations: GI, gastrointestinal; ECF, extracellular fluid; GFR, glomerular filtration rate

TABLE 7–11: Cl⁻-Resistant Metabolic Alkalosis with Hypertension (Elevated Aldosterone Levels)

Renal artery stenosis

The most common cause of Cl^--resistant metabolic alkalosis with associated hypertension is renovascular disease

Renal artery stenosis is a frequent clinical problem that develops in the elderly and those with advanced atherosclerotic disease

Primary aldosteronism

Excess aldosterone acts as both the initiation and maintenance factor for metabolic alkalosis

Increased H^+ secretion promotes reclamation of filtered HCO_3^- in proximal tubule and generation of new HCO_3^- in distal nephron that is ultimately retained in the ECF

Although increased ECF volume tends to mitigate the alkalosis by decreasing proximal tubular bicarbonate reabsorption, distal processes aid in maintenance of an elevated plasma HCO_3^- threshold

Primary aldosteronism may be caused by an adrenal tumor, which selectively synthesizes aldosterone (Conn's syndrome) or hyperplasia (usually bilateral) of the adrenal cortex

Diagnosis of a primary mineralocorticoid excess state depends on the demonstration that ECF volume is expanded (e.g., nonstimulatible plasma renin activity) and nonsuppressible aldosterone secretion is present (e.g., demonstration that exogenous mineralocorticoids and high salt diet or acute volume expansion with saline do not suppress plasma aldosterone concentration)

Recent data suggest that primary aldosteronism may occur in as many as 8% of adult hypertensive patients; many of these patients do not have a significant metabolic alkalosis

Abbreviation: ECF, extracellular fluid

TABLE 7–12: Diagnosis of Primary Aldosteronism

The diagnosis of primary aldosteronism generally involves three phases—a screening test, the confirmation of nonsuppressible aldosterone secretion, and finally subtype differentiation

Plasma aldosterone to renin ratio (ARR)—screening

The most common screening test employed

Serum potassium concentration should be normal

Highly dependent on the value of the denominator—plasma renin concentration; the lower limit of detection in an individual laboratory is very important

Aldosterone antagonists (spironolactone or eplerenone) and high dose amiloride (> 5mg/day) must be stopped for 6–8 weeks

ACE inhibitors, ARBs, β blockers and calcium channel blockers may falsely lower the ratio

The ARR cutoff varies depending on the circumstances of the test; the cutoff values are: (1) 0900 sample after lying in bed overnight–35; (2) 1300 sample after 4 h of ambulation–13.1; (3) seated prior to saline load test–23.6; (4) seated post saline load–18.5. A plasma aldosterone concentration greater than 15 ng/dL has also been added to the ARR criteria by some authors

Confirm nonsuppressible aldosterone secretion

Oral salt loading test

- Five gram sodium diet for 3 days

- Caution must be used in severely hypertensive patients, renal K^+ excretion may increase and serum K^+ must be monitored closely

TABLE 7–12 (Continued)
• On the third day collect a 24-h urine for Na^+, creatinine and aldosterone
• Urinary Na^+ must be > 200 mEq/day to document Na^+ loading and urinary aldosterone should suppress to < 12 $\mu g/24$ h in normals
Saline suppression test
• Administer 2 L of normal saline over 2 h with the patient sitting
• The plasma aldosterone concentration should decline to < 5 ng/dL in normals
Differentiation of aldosterone-producing adenoma from idiopathic bilateral adrenal hyperplasia
CT or MRI
• Unilateral mass > 4 cm suggestive of adrenal carcinoma
• Absence of a mass does not exclude an adenoma
• Presence of a mass does not rule out bilateral adrenal hyperplasia except perhaps in the young patient
Adrenal vein sampling
• The gold standard test
• Technically difficult and can be complicated by adrenal hemorrhage or adrenal vein dissection
• Not required in patients ≤ age 40 with plasma aldosterone concentrations ≥ 30 ng/dL and a > 1 cm hypodense adrenal mass (< 10 Hounsfield units) on CT

(continued)

TABLE 7–12 (Continued)
• Cortisol is also sampled to verify catheter placement in adrenal veins
• Unilateral adenomas are detected by examining the aldosterone ratio on each side before and after the administration of ACTH. A ratio greater than 3 (affected/unaffected side) is indicative of an adenoma
Abbreviations: ARR, aldosterone to renin ratio; ACE, angiotensin converting enzyme; ARB, angiotensin receptor blocker; CT, computed tomography; MRI, magnetic resonance imaging; ACTH, adrenocorticotrophic hormone

TABLE 7–13: Cl^--Resistant Metabolic Alkalosis—with Hypertension (Suppressed Aldosterone Levels-Acquired Disorders)
In this group of disorders glucocorticoids or genetic defects mimic aldosterone action in collecting duct; resulting volume expansion suppresses renin and aldosterone
Cushing's syndrome
Characterized by excessive corticosteroid synthesis
Tumors that secrete ectopic ACTH are more likely to cause hypokalemia and metabolic alkalosis than pituitary tumors
Most corticosteroids (specifically cortisol, deoxycorticosterone, and corticosterone) also have significant mineralocorticoid effects and produce hypokalemic metabolic alkalosis

TABLE 7–13 (Continued)
Collecting duct cells contain type II 11β-HSD that degrades cortisol to the inactive metabolite cortisone; cortisol secretion in response to ectopic ACTH may be so high, however, that it overwhelms the metabolic capacity of the enzyme; in addition, type II 11β-HSD may be inhibited by ACTH
Licorice
Glycyrrhizic and glycyrrhetinic acid, which are found in both licorice and chewing tobacco, may cause a hypokalemic metabolic alkalosis accompanied by hypertension, and thus, simulate primary aldosteronism
This chemical inhibits type II 11β-hydroxysteroid dehydrogenase activity and "uncovers" the mineralocorticoid receptor which is normally "protected" by this enzyme from glucocorticoid stimulation
Glucocorticoids produce comparable stimulation of the mineralocorticoid receptor and result in a clinical syndrome similar to primary aldosteronism without elevated plasma aldosterone concentration
Abbreviations: ACTH, adrenocorticotropic hormone; HSD, hydroxysteroid dehydrogenase

TABLE 7–14: Evaluation of the Patient with Suspected Cushing's Syndrome

After a careful history to exclude all sources of exogenous glucocorticoids the evaluation of Cushing's syndrome proceeds through three stages. It should be recognized that there is little consensus as to which tests are best at each stage

Step 1 Is Cushing's syndrome present?

24 h urinary free cortisol-values greater than 3 times the ULN are highly sensitive and specific. Values between ULN and 3 times ULN require repeat testing and clinical judgment depending on the level of suspicion

Overnight dexamethasone suppression test-One mg given between 11 PM and midnight followed by an 8 AM serum cortisol. Serum cortisol should suppress to < 1.8 µg/dL in normals

Late evening salivary cortisol less than 1.3 ng/mL in normals; this test is becoming increasingly popular because of its ease of collection and stability of cortisol in saliva at room temperature

False positives for these tests include obesity, chronic illness, alcoholism, and depression

Is Cushing's syndrome a result of an ACTH-independent (primary adrenal disease) or ACTH-dependent (pituitary adenoma or ectopic tumor production) process?

Late night plasma ACTH and cortisol (11 PM-midnight)-Serum cortisol should be > 15µg/dL; ACTH < 10 pg/ml-ACTH-independent process, ACTH > 20 pg/ml ACTH-dependent process

TABLE 7–14 (Continued)

Indeterminant values require more sophisticated testing

ACTH-independent disease should be further examined with either an adrenal CT or MRI

Differentiating the causes of ACTH-dependent disease

High dose dexamethasone suppression test-2mg every 6 h with 24 h urines collected for free cortisol and 17-hydroxysteroids; suppression is compatible with a pituitary adenoma; free cortisol should suppress > 90% and 17-hydroxysteroids > 64% compared to baseline; lack of suppression is indicative of ectopic ACTH production and can be further evaluated with an octreotide scan or MRI

Patients with ectopic ACTH production often have severe hypokalemia and metabolic alkalosis

Abbreviations: ULN, upper limit of normal; ACTH, adrenocorticotrophic hormone; CT, computed tomography; MRI, magnetic resonance imaging

TABLE 7–15: Cl⁻-Resistant Metabolic Alkalosis—with Hypertension (Suppressed Aldosterone Levels-Inherited Disorders)

GRA

Most common monogenic disorder associated with severe early onset hypertension

Develops from a gene duplication fusing regulatory sequences of an isoform of the 11β-hydroxylase gene to the coding sequence of the aldosterone synthase gene

Diagnosis should be entertained in those whose family members also have difficult to control hypertension

Clinical confirmation is pursued with the measurement of elevated concentrations of 18-OH-cortisol and 18-oxotetrahydrocortisol in urine prior to genetic analysis

Patients with GRA can often be successfully treated with low dose glucocorticoid supplementation (0.25–0.50 mg dexamethasone/day)

Liddle's syndrome

A rare autosomal dominant disorder resulting from a mutation in either the β- or γ-subunit of the Na^+ channel expressed in the apical membrane of the collecting duct

The mutation increases Na^+ reabsorption by blocking channel removal from the membrane

Metabolic alkalosis, hypokalemia, and severe hypertension are characteristic

No blood pressure response to spironolactone

TABLE 7–15 (Continued)

Apparent mineralocorticoid excess

Autosomal recessive

Loss of function mutations in type II 11β-HSD

Presents with severe early onset hypertension and hypokalemia

Clinical confirmation is pursued with the measurement of elevated tetrahydrocortisol concentrations and an elevated allotetrahydrocortisol to tetrahydrocortisol ratio in urine prior to genetic analysis

Congenital adrenal hyperplasia

Results from a hereditary deficiency in several enzymes involved in cortisol biosynthesis (Figure 7–4); most are associated with salt wasting, hypotension, and hyperkalemia

11β hydroxylase deficiency—5–8% of cases

Autosomal recessive

Associated with hypertension, metabolic alkalosis, androgen excess, and virilization

Elevated levels of 11-deoxycortisol and 11-deoxycorticosterone

Abbreviations: GRA, glucorticoid remediable aldosteronism; HSD, hydroxysteroid dehydrogenase

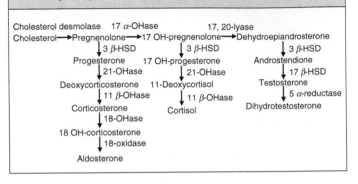

FIGURE 7–4: Steroid Biosynthesis Pathway.
HSD-Hydroxysteroid dehydrogenase, OHase-Hydroxylase

TABLE 7–16: Cl^--Resistant Metabolic Alkalosis— without Hypertension

Bartter syndrome

Characterized by hyperreninemia, hyperaldosteronemia in the absence of hypertension or Na^+ retention

This rare condition generally presents in childhood and is caused by defects in one of five genes that are involved in thick ascending limb Cl^- transport (see Figure 7–4): the apical Na^+-K^+-$2Cl^-$ transporter; the ROMK channel; the basolateral Cl^- channel (CLC-K_b); the β-subunit of the basolateral Cl^- channel (Barrtin); or a gain of function mutation in the Ca^{2+}-sensing receptor

These defects result in high distal nephron Na^+ and Cl^- delivery, RAAS activation, and development of hypokalemic metabolic alkalosis

Gitelman's syndrome

Caused by mutations in the thiazide-sensitive NaCl transporter in the distal convoluted tubule

Presents in adulthood and is more common than Bartter syndrome

Bartter and Gitelman's syndromes can closely mimic diuretic abuse; they can be functionally imitated by the pharmacologic administration of loop and thiazide diuretics, respectively; it is important to consider surreptitious diuretic use as an alternative to these diagnoses, especially if patients present as adolescents or adults with previously normal serum K^+ and bicarbonate concentrations

(continued)

TABLE 7–16 (Continued)

Measuring diuretic concentrations in urine is often part of the initial workup

Profound K$^+$ depletion

Severe hypokalemia (serum [K$^+$] < 2 mEq/L) may sometimes convert a Cl$^-$-responsive to a Cl$^-$-resistant metabolic alkalosis

In some reports, affected individuals did not demonstrate mineralocorticoid excess, and their alkalosis did not correct with Na$^+$ repletion until K$^+$ was repleted

Hypercalcemia (nonhyperparathyroid etiology)

Patients with hypercalcemia from malignancy or sarcoid, and not from hyperparathyroidism, may develop a mild metabolic alkalosis

This is likely to be due to the Ca^{2+}-mediated suppression of PTH, which may raise the PT for HCO$_3^-$ reabsorption

Poststarvation

After a prolonged fast, administration of carbohydrates may produce a metabolic alkalosis that persists for weeks

The initiation factor is not known, but increased renal Na$^+$ reabsorption secondary to ECF volume depletion is responsible for maintenance of the alkalosis

Abbreviations: RAAS, renin-angiotensin-aldosterone system; PTH, parathyroid hormone; PT, plasma threshold; ECF, extracellular fluid

FIGURE 7–5: Cell Model of the Thick Ascending Limb

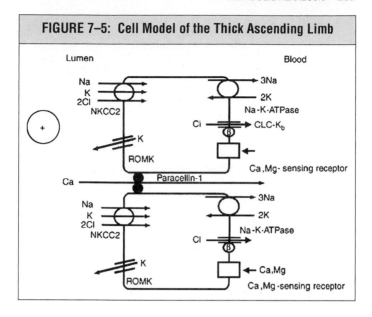

TABLE 7–17: Approach to the Patient with Cl⁻-Resistant Metabolic Alkalosis

Patients are initially subdivided based on the presence or absence of hypertension; those patients with hypertension can then be further categorized based on their renin and aldosterone concentrations

Disorder	Renin Concentration	Aldosterone Concentration
Primary aldosteronism	Decreased	Increased
Renal artery stenosis	Increased	Increased
Renin-producing tumor	Increased	Increased
Cushing's syndrome	Decreased	Decreased
Licorice ingestion	Decreased	Decreased
Apparent mineralocorti-coid excess	Decreased	Decreased
Liddle's syndrome	Decreased	Decreased

TREATMENT

TABLE 7–18: Treatment
Treatment of metabolic alkalosis, as with all acid-base disturbances, hinges on correction of the underlying disease state
The severity of the acid-base disturbance itself may be life threatening in some cases, and require specific therapy; this is especially true in mixed acid-base disturbances where pH changes are in the same direction (such as a respiratory alkalosis from sepsis and a metabolic alkalosis secondary to vomiting)
Emergent control of systemic pH
In the setting of a clinical emergency, controlled hypoventilation must be employed
In this clinical condition, intubation, sedation, and controlled hypoventilation with a mechanical ventilator (sometimes using inspired CO_2 and/or supplemental oxygen to prevent hypoxia) is often lifesaving
Urgent control of systemic pH
Once the situation is no longer critical, partial or complete correction of metabolic alkalosis over the ensuing 6–8 h with HCl administered as a 0.15-M solution through a central vein is preferred; arginine hydrochloride can also be used
The effect of HCl is not rapid enough to prevent or treat life-threatening complications

(continued)

TABLE 7–18 (Continued)

Generally, the "acid deficit" is calculated assuming a bicarbonate distribution space of 0.5 times body weight in liters, and about half of this amount of HCl is given with frequent monitoring of blood gases and electrolytes

These agents can result in significant potential complications; hydrochloric acid may cause intravascular hemolysis and tissue necrosis, while ammonium chloride may result in ammonia toxicity

Noncritical situations

In less urgent settings, metabolic alkalosis is treated after examining whether it is Cl^--responsive or not

Cl^--responsive metabolic alkalosis is responsive to volume repletion; coexistent hypokalemia should also be corrected

Cl^--resistant metabolic alkaloses are treated by antagonizing the mineralocorticoid (or mineralocorticoid-like substance) that maintains renal H^+ losses; this sometimes can be accomplished with spironolactone, eplerenone, or other distal K^+-sparing diuretics like amiloride

It is not unusual that the cause of metabolic alkalosis is due to a therapy that is essential in the management of a disease state

- The proximal tubule diuretic acetazolamide, which decreases the PT for HCO_3^- by inhibiting proximal tubule HCO_3^- reabsorption, may need to be added to the diuretic regimen of patient's with severe edema forming states

- Prescription of a proton pump inhibitor will decrease gastric H^+ losses in the patient who requires prolonged gastric drainage

Abbreviation: PT, plasma threshold

8

Respiratory and Mixed
Acid-Base Disturbances

RESPIRATORY DISTURBANCES

TABLE 8–1: Introduction
Definitions
Breathing—an automatic, rhythmic, and centrally regulated process by which contraction of the diaphragm and rib cage moves gas in and out of airways and alveolae of the lung
Respiration—includes breathing, but also involves the circulation of blood, allowing for O_2 intake and CO_2 excretion
Control of breathing
Automatic
• Largely under the control of PCO_2
• Control center resides in the brainstem within the reticular activating system (medullary respiratory areas and pontine respiratory group)
Volitional—less is known about this control mechanism

FIGURE 8–1: A Simplified Schematic of Elements Involved in Controlling Ventilation

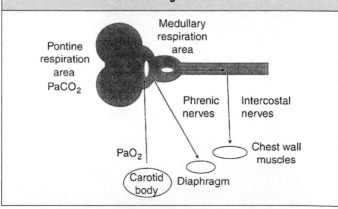

Pontine respiration area
PaCO$_2$

Medullary respiration area

Phrenic nerves

Intercostal nerves

Chest wall muscles

PaO$_2$

Carotid body

Diaphragm

TABLE 8–2: Chemoreceptors and the Control of Automatic Breathing

The two systems (central and peripheral) interact, with hypoxia the central response to PCO_2 is enhanced

Central

Located in the medulla of the CNS

Responds to changes in $PaCO_2$ largely through changes in brain pH (interstitial and cytosolic)

A sensitive system, $PaCO_2$ control is generally tight

Respiratory control by oxygen tensions is much less important until PaO_2 falls to levels below 70 mmHg; this is a reflection of the Hb-O_2 dissociation curve since Hb saturation is generally above 94% until PaO_2 falls below 70 mmHg

Peripheral

Located in the carotid bodies although less important receptors were identified in the aortic arch

O_2 control of respiration is mediated largely through peripheral chemoreceptors which, in response to low PaO_2, close ATP-sensitive K^+ channels and depolarize glomus cells in the carotid body

With chronic hypercapnia, control of respiration by CO_2 is severely blunted leaving some patients' respiration almost entirely under the control of O_2 tensions

Abbreviations: CNS, central nervous system; ATP, adenosine triphosphate

TABLE 8–3: The Physical Machinery of Breathing

Involves both the lungs, as well as bones and thoracic musculature that interact to move air in and out of the pulmonary air spaces

Abnormalities of either the skeleton, musculature, or airways, air spaces, and lung blood supply may impair respiration

The physical machinery of breathing can be assessed by PFTs

PFTs readily differentiate problems with airway resistance (e.g., asthma or COPD) from those of alveolar diffusion (e.g., interstitial fibrosis) or neuromuscular function (e.g., phrenic nerve palsy, Guillian-Barré syndrome)

Pulmonary ventilation—the amount of gas brought into and/or out of the lung

Expressed as minute ventilation (i.e., how much air is inspired and expired within 1 min) or in functional terms as alveolar ventilation since the portion of ventilation confined to conductance airways does not effectively exchange O_2 for CO_2 in alveolae

We can reference ventilation with regard to either O_2 or CO_2, however, since CO_2 excretion is so effective and ambient CO_2 tensions in the atmosphere are low, pulmonary ventilation generally is synonymous with pulmonary CO_2 excretion

CO_2 is much more soluble than O_2 and exchange across the alveolar capillary for CO_2 is essentially complete under most circumstances, whereas some O_2 gradient from alveolus to the alveolar capillary is always present

Abbreviations: PFT, pulmonary function test; COPD, chronic obstructive pulmonary disease

RESPIRATORY ACIDOSIS

Defined as a primary increase in $PaCO_2$ secondary to decreased effective ventilation with net CO_2 retention.

This decrease in effective ventilation can occur from defects in any aspect of ventilation control or implementation.

TABLE 8–4: Causes of Respiratory Acidosis
Acute
Airway obstruction—aspiration of foreign body or vomitus, laryngospasm, generalized bronchospasm, obstructive sleep apnea
Respiratory center depression—general anesthesia, sedative overdosage, cerebral trauma or infarction, central sleep apnea
Circulatory catastrophes—cardiac arrest, severe pulmonary edema
Neuromuscular defects—high cervical cordotomy, botulism, tetanus, Guillain-Barré syndrome, crisis in myasthenia gravis, familial hypokalemic periodic paralysis, hypokalemic myopathy, toxic drug agents (e.g., curare, succinylcholine, aminoglycosides, organophosphates)
Restrictive defects—pneumothorax, hemothorax, flail chest, severe pneumonitis, hyaline membrane disease, adult respiratory distress syndrome
Pulmonary disorders—pneumonia, massive pulmonary embolism, pulmonary edema
Mechanical underventilation

TABLE 8–4 (Continued)

Chronic

Airway obstruction—chronic obstructive lung disease (bronchitis, emphysema)

Respiratory center depression—chronic sedative depression, primary alveolar hypoventilation, obesity hypoventilation syndrome, brain tumor, bulbar poliomyelitis

Neuromuscular defects—poliomyelitis, multiple sclerosis, muscular dystrophy, amyotrophic lateral sclerosis, diaphragmatic paralysis, myxedema, myopathic disease (e.g., polymyositis, acid maltase deficiency)

Restrictive defects—kyphoscoliosis, spinal arthritis, fibrothorax, hydrothorax, interstitial fibrosis, decreased diaphragmatic movement (e.g., ascites), prolonged pneumonitis, obesity

TABLE 8–5: Compensation for Respiratory Acidosis

Compensation for respiratory acidosis occurs at several levels; some of these processes are rapid, whereas others are slower; this latter fact allows us to distinguish between acute and chronic respiratory acidosis in some cases

With respiratory acidosis, a rise in $[HCO_3^-]$ is a normal, compensatory response

As is the case for metabolic disorders, a failure of this normal adaptive response is indicative of the presence of metabolic acidosis in the setting of a complex or mixed acid-base disturbance

Conversely, an exaggerated increase in HCO_3^- producing a normal pH indicates the presence of metabolic alkalosis in the setting of a complex or mixed acid-base disturbance

Mechanisms

Acute

Increases in $PaCO_2$ and decreases in O_2 tension stimulate ventilatory drive

Increases in $PaCO_2$ are immediately accompanied by a shift to the right of the reaction shown below in Eq. (8-1) resulting in an increase in HCO_3^- concentration

$[HCO_3^-]$ in mEq/L increases by 0.1 times the increase in $PaCO_2$ in mmHg (±2 mEq/L)

Chronic

The kidney provides the mechanism for the majority of chronic compensation

TABLE 8–5 (Continued)

As $PaCO_2$ increases and arterial pH decreases, renal acid excretion and bicarbonate retention become more avid; some of this is a direct chemical consequence of elevated $PaCO_2$ and mass action facilitating intracellular bicarbonate formation, whereas other portions involve genomic adaptations of tubular cells involved in renal acid excretion

Enzymes involved in renal ammoniagenesis (e.g., glutamine synthetase), as well as apical and basolateral ion transport proteins (e.g., Na^+-H^+ exchanger, Na^+-K^+ ATPase) are synthesized in increased amounts at key sites within the nephron

Chronic respiratory acidosis present for at least 4–5 days is accompanied by a $[HCO_3^-]$ increase = 0.4 times the increase in $PaCO_2$ (mmHg) ($\pm$3 mEq/L)

Renal correction never completely returns arterial pH to the level it was at prior to CO_2 retention

$$H_2CO_3 \rightarrow H^- + HCO_3^- \qquad (8\text{-}1)$$

Abbreviation: ATP, adenosine triphosphate

RESPIRATORY ALKALOSIS

Respiratory alkalosis is defined as a primary decrease in $PaCO_2$ secondary to an increase in effective ventilation with net CO_2 removal. This increase in effective ventilation can occur from defects in any aspect of ventilation control or implementation.

TABLE 8–6: Causes of Respiratory Alkalosis
Hypoxia
Decreased inspired oxygen tension
Ventilation-perfusion inequality
Hypotension
Severe anemia
CNS mediated
Voluntary hyperventilation
Neurologic disease: cerebrovascular accident (infarction; hemorrhage); infection (encephalitis, meningitis); trauma; tumor
Pharmacologic and hormonal stimulation—salicylates, ditrophenol, nicotine, xanthines, pressor hormones, pregnancy
Pulmonary disease
Interstitial lung disease
Pneumonia
Pulmonary embolism

TABLE 8–6 (Continued)
Pulmonary edema
Mechanical overventilation
Miscellaneous
Hepatic failure
Gram-negative septicemia
Anxiety-hyperventilation syndrome
Heat exposure
Abbreviation: CNS, central nervous system

TABLE 8–7: Compensation for Respiratory Alkalosis

The normal compensatory response is a fall in $[HCO_3^-]$

Failure of this normal adaptive response is indicative of the presence of metabolic alkalosis in the setting of a complex or mixed acid-base disturbance

An exaggerated decrease in $[HCO_3^-]$ producing a normal pH indicates the presence of metabolic acidosis in the setting of a complex or mixed acid-base disturbance

Mechanisms

• Acute

Decreases in $PaCO_2$ will inhibit ventilatory drive, in some way antagonizing the process that led to reductions in CO_2 tension

Decreases in $PaCO_2$ are immediately accompanied by a shift to the left of the reaction shown in Eq. (8-1) and decreases in $[HCO_3^-]$ result

The decrease in $[HCO_3^-]$ (in mEq/L) is 0.1 times the decrease in $PaCO_2$ in mmHg (with an error range of ±2 mEq/L)

• Chronic

The kidney provides the mechanism for the majority of chronic compensation

As $PaCO_2$ decreases and arterial pH increases, renal excretion of acid and retention of bicarbonate are reduced

TABLE 8–7 (Continued)

Chronic respiratory alkalosis present for at least 4–5 days will be accompanied by a $[HCO_3^-]$ decrease (in mEq/L) of 0.4 times the increase in $PaCO_2$ (mmHg) (with an error range of ±3 mEq/L)

Renal correction never completely returns arterial pH to the level it was at prior to respiratory alkalosis

Decreases in $[HCO_3^-]$ below 12 mEq/L are generally not seen from metabolic compensation for respiratory alkalosis

MIXED DISTURBANCES

TABLE 8–8: The Diagnosis of Mixed Disturbances—Degree of Compensation
One first evaluates the degree of compensation
Inadequate compensation is equivalent to another primary acid-base disturbance
It is important to recognize that compensation is never complete; compensatory processes cannot return one's blood pH to what it was before one suffered a primary disturbance
The first clue to the presence of a mixed acid-base disorder is the degree of compensation, "over compensation" or an absence of compensation are certain indicators that a mixed acid-base disorder is present
For metabolic disorders, respiratory compensation should be immediate; it is relatively easy to determine whether compensation is appropriate using the rules of compensation below
Rules of compensation-metabolic disturbances
• Metabolic acidosis: compensatory change in $PaCO_2$ (mmHg) = 1–1.5 × the fall in $[HCO_3^-]$ (mEq/L) or the $PaCO_2$ (mmHg) = 1.5 × $[HCO_3^-]$ + 8 ± 2
• Metabolic alkalosis: compensatory change in $PaCO_2$ (mmHg) = 0.6 – 1 × the increase in $[HCO_3^-]$ (mEq/L)

TABLE 8–8 (Continued)

For respiratory disorders metabolic compensation takes days to become complete; mass action will produce about a 0.1 mEq/L change in [HCO_3^-] for every 1 mmHg change in $PaCO_2$; a complete absence of metabolic compensation for respiratory acidosis or alkalosis clearly indicates a second primary disturbance; for degrees of compensation between 0.1 and 0.4 mEq/L/mmHg change in $PaCO_2$, it is difficult if not impossible to distinguish between a failure of compensation (e.g., a primary metabolic disorder) and an acute respiratory disturbance on the blood gas alone

Rules of compensation-respiratory disturbances

- Acute respiratory acidosis or alkalosis: compensatory change in [HCO_3^-] (mEq/L) = 0.1 × the change in $PaCO_2$ (mmHg) ± 2 (mEq/L)

- Chronic respiratory acidosis or alkalosis: compensatory change in [HCO_3^-] (mEq/L) = 0.4 × the change in $PaCO_2$ (mmHg) ± 3 (mEq/L)

TABLE 8–9: The Diagnosis of Mixed Disturbances— the Search for Hidden Disorders

One next evaluates the anion gap (Eq. 8-2)
Calculating the SAG provides insight into the differential diagnosis of metabolic acidosis (anion gap and nonanion gap metabolic acidosis) and can also indicate that metabolic acidosis is present in the patient with an associated metabolic alkalosis
Compare the change in SAG to the change in serum bicarbonate concentration; if the change in the SAG is much larger than the fall in serum bicarbonate concentration, one can infer the presence of both an anion gap metabolic acidosis and metabolic alkalosis
If the fall in serum bicarbonate concentration is; however, much larger than the increase in the SAG (and the SAG is significantly increased) one can infer the presence of both an anion gap and nonanion gap metabolic acidosis
$$\mathbf{SAG} = [Na^+] - [Cl^-] - [HCO_3^-] \qquad (8\text{-}2)$$ Formula for the serum anion gap (SAG)
Abbreviation: SAG, serum anion gap

FIGURE 8–2: Use of the Anion Gap in Evaluation of Mixed Acid-Base Disturbances. To use the SAG in the approach to a complex acid-base disorder, we make the stoichiometric assumption that for a pure organic acidosis $\Delta SAG = \Delta[HCO_3^-]$. Since we don't have "pre" and "post" disorder values, we further assume that SAG started at 10 mEq/L and $[HCO_3^-]$ started at 24 mEq/L. With these assumptions, we can diagnose simultaneous anion gap metabolic acidosis and metabolic alkalosis when the SAG is large and the decrease in $[HCO_3^-]$ is relatively small. Conversely, we can Also diagnose simultaneous nonanion gap metabolic acidosis with anion gap metabolic acidosis if the fall in $[HCO_3^-]$ is much larger than the modestly but significantly increased SAG

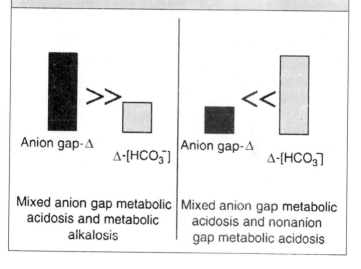

Anion gap-Δ Δ-$[HCO_3^-]$ Anion gap-Δ Δ-$[HCO_3^-]$

Mixed anion gap metabolic acidosis and metabolic alkalosis | Mixed anion gap metabolic acidosis and nonanion gap metabolic acidosis

FIGURE 8–3: Acid-Base Nomogram. A second approach to the evaluation of mixed acid-base disturbances involves the use of a nomogram rather than using the rules of compensation and the interpretation of the serum anion gap

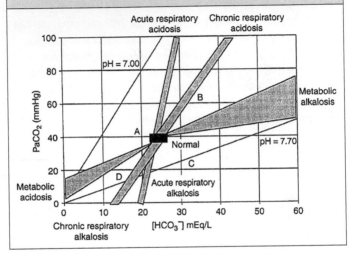

TABLE 8–10: Syndromes Commonly Associated with Mixed Acid-Base Disorders

Hemodynamic compromise

Cardiopulmonary arrest

Pulmonary edema

Sepsis

Liver failure

Poisonings

Ethylene glycol intoxication

Methanol intoxication

Aspirin intoxication

Ethanol intoxication

Metabolic disturbances

Severe hypokalemia

Severe hypophosphatemia

Diabetic ketoacidosis

Bowel ischemia

COPD

Chronic kidney disease

Abbreviation: COPD, chronic obstructive pulmonary disease

TABLE 8–11: The Importance of the Diagnosis of Mixed Acid-Base Disorders

Helps one gain insight into the clinical problems the patient is facing

Confers appropriate urgency to the clinical situation

Prompts a search for potential causes of additional acid-base disturbance(s)

Treatment of the acid-base disorder always involves making the correct clinical diagnosis of the underlying causes and appropriate specific therapy directed at those causes

9
Disorders of Serum Calcium

REGULATION

TABLE 9–1: Regulation of ECF Ionized Calcium
Only a small percentage of total body Ca^{2+} is in the ECF
• This is the fraction that is physiologically regulated
Regulation is via PTH, the Ca^{2+}-sensing receptor and calcitriol action in parathyroid gland, bone, intestine, and kidney
Calcium fractions in blood
• Sixty percent of calcium is ultrafilterable and is either ionized and free in solution (50%) or complexed to anions (10%)
• Forty percent is bound to albumin
The majority of total body Ca^{2+} exists as hydroxyapatite in bone (99%)
• The bone Ca^{2+} reservoir is so large that one cannot become hypocalcemic without a decrease in bone Ca^{2+} release due to a defect in either PTH or calcitriol action
Abbreviations: ECF, extracellular fluid; PTH, parathyroid hormone

TABLE 9–2: Calcium Fluxes between ECF and Organ Systems

The average adult takes in 1000 mg of Ca^{2+}/day

Twenty percent is absorbed in intestine

In the steady state intestinal absorption is matched by urinary excretion

The kidney excretes approximately 2% (200 mg) of the filtered Ca^{2+} load

Abbreviation: ECF, extracellular fluid

FIGURE 9–1: Total Body Calcium Homeostasis

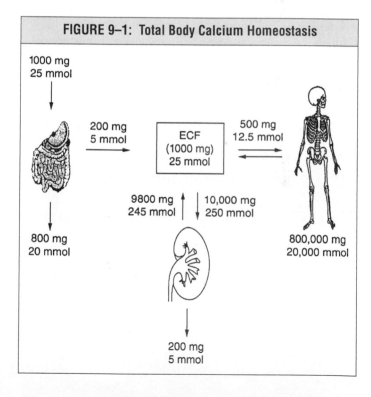

TABLE 9–3: The Calcium–Sensing Receptor

Expression

Plasma membrane of parathyroid gland

- Couples changes in ECF Ca^{2+} concentration to the regulation of PTH secretion (Figure 9–2)

- Mediated via several signaling pathways (phospholipase A2, C, D, and other pathways)

Expressed on the cell surface in kidney, lung, intestine, and a variety of other organs

Ca^{2+}-sensing receptor knockout mice demonstrate marked parathyroid hyperplasia suggesting that the receptor also plays a role in parathyroid cell growth and proliferation

Systemic actions

High Ca^{2+} concentration activates the receptor and inhibits PTH release

Low Ca^{2+} concentrations stimulate PTH secretion and production, and increase parathyroid gland mass

This system responds within minutes to changes in Ca^{2+} concentration

The parathyroid gland does not contain a large supply of excess PTH storage granules

Basal and stimulated PTH secretion can only be supported for a few hours in the absence of new hormone synthesis

There is an inverse sigmoidal relationship between Ca^{2+} concentration and PTH secretion (Figure 9–2)

TABLE 9–3 (Continued)

Actions in kidney

Thick ascending limb—expressed in the basolateral membrane

- Arachidonic acid intermediates inhibit K^+ recycling (responsible for the lumen-positive voltage)

- The lumen-positive voltage is the driving force for paracellular Ca^{2+} transport—urinary Ca^{2+} excretion increases with receptor activation

Inner medullary collecting duct—expressed in the apical membrane

- Receptor activation impairs concentrating ability

- The receptor is present in the apical membrane in the same vesicles that contain water channels

- Perfusion of the inner medullary collecting duct with a high Ca^{2+} solution reduces vasopressin-stimulated water flow by about 40% presumably via activation of the receptor

- May provide a mechanism to inhibit Ca^{2+} crystallization in states of hypercalciuria

- Inhibition of water transport may aid in increasing the solubility of Ca^{2+} salts

Abbreviations: ECF, extracellular fluid; PTH, parathyroid hormone

FIGURE 9–2: Relationship between PTH Released by Parathyroid Gland and ECF Ionized Ca^{2+} Concentration. As can be seen in the figure, there is still some basal PTH secretion even at high Ca^{2+} concentrations. This is important clinically in the patient with secondary hyperparathyroidism and end-stage renal disease. As parathyroid gland mass increases basal PTH secretion increases to the point where it can no longer be suppressed by high dose calcitriol therapy and ultimately subtotal parathyroidectomy is required

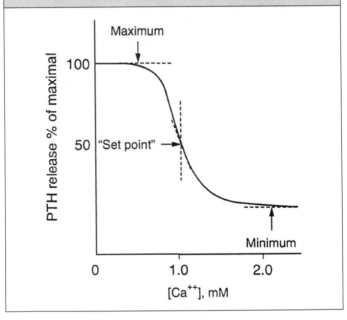

TABLE 9–4: PTH Mechanisms of Action

PTH increases ECF Ca^{2+} concentration via effects in bone, intestine, and kidney—the end result is an increase in ECF Ca^{2+} concentration without an increase in phosphorus concentration

Bone

- In the presence of calcitriol, PTH stimulates bone resorption via an increase in osteoclast number and activity

Intestine

- Acts indirectly through stimulation of calcitriol formation to increase Ca^{2+} and phosphorus absorption

- Increases epithelial Ca^{2+} channel expression in intestine

Kidney

- Increases Ca^{2+} reabsorption in distal convoluted tubule and connecting tubule

- Stimulates activity of 1-α-hydroxylase in the proximal convoluted tubule that converts 25(OH) vitamin D_3 to 1, 25 $(OH)_2$ vitamin D_3

- Reduces proximal tubular reabsorption of phosphate and bicarbonate

Abbreviations: ECF, extracellular fluid; PTH, parathyroid hormone

FIGURE 9–3: The Calcitriol Biosynthetic Pathway.
7-Dehydrocholesterol in skin is converted to vitamin D_3 by UV light. Vitamin D_3 is then 25 hydroxylated in liver. This step is poorly regulated and in general 25(OH) vitamin D_3 concentration parallels vitamin D intake. Finally, 1-α-hydroxylation takes place in the inner mitochondrial membrane of proximal tubular cells. Increasing PTH concentration and hypophosphatemia enhance 1-α-hydroxylase activity. Calcitriol stimulates its own catabolism via activation of 24 hydroxylase. Twenty-Four hydroxylase is the major catabolic enzyme in calcitriol target tissues. It is upregulated by calcitriol, hypercalcemia, and hyperphosphatemia

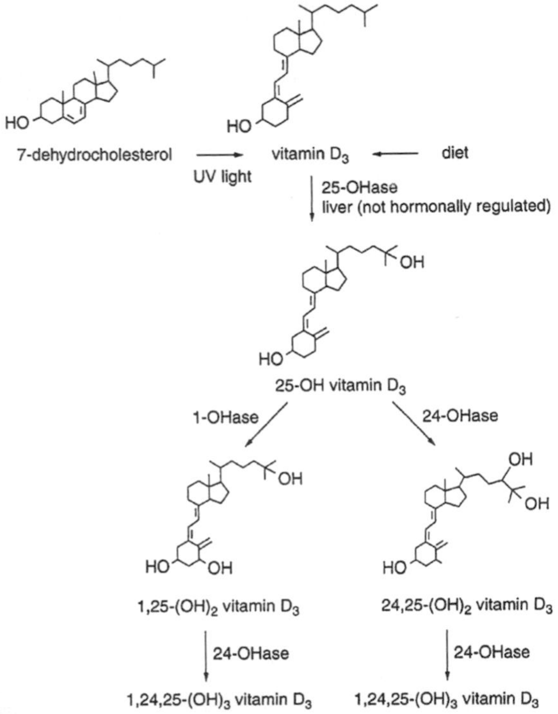

TABLE 9–5: Calcitriol
Increases Ca^{2+} and phosphorus availability for bone formation and prevents hypocalcemia and hypophosphatemia
In intestine and kidney, calcitriol stimulates Ca^{2+} transport via upregulating the expression of Ca^{2+}-binding proteins (calbindins)
• Calbindins bind Ca^{2+} and move it from the apical to the basolateral membrane, thereby allowing Ca^{2+} to move through the cell without an increase in free intracellular Ca^{2+} concentration
Increases expression of the Na^{+}-phosphate cotransporter in intestine
In bone calcitriol has a variety of effects: (1) potentiation of PTH effects; (2) stimulation of osteoclastic reabsorption; and (3) induction of monocyte differentiation into osteoclasts
In parathyroid gland calcitriol binds its receptor in the cytoplasm and forms a heterodimer with the retinoid X receptor and is translocated to the nucleus
• The complex binds to the PTH gene promoter and decreases PTH expression, as well as inhibits parathyroid growth
Abbreviation: PTH, parathyroid hormone

TABLE 9–6: Renal Calcium Excretion

Ca^{2+} that is not bound to albumin is freely filtered at the glomerulus

Proximal tubule

- Reabsorbs two-thirds of the filtered Ca^{2+} load

- Majority of reabsorption is passive but there is a small active component

- Ca^{2+} transport parallels that of Na^+ and water

- Ca^{2+} reabsorption proximally varies directly with ECF volume

- The more expanded ECF volume—the higher urinary Ca^{2+} excretion

- Urinary Ca^{2+} excretion is decreased in the setting of volume contraction

Thick ascending limb

- Reabsorbs 25% of the filtered Ca^{2+} load

- Ca^{2+} transport is passive, paracellular, and depends on the magnitude of the lumen-positive transepithelial voltage

- The lumen-positive voltage is the result of K^+ recycling across the apical membrane via a K^+ channel (ROMK)

- Dissipation of the voltage eliminates the driving force for Ca^{2+} reabsorption and increases urinary Ca^{2+} excretion

- Loop diuretics (furosemide) block the Na^+-K^+-$2Cl^-$ cotransporter, dissipate the voltage gradient, and increase Ca^{2+} excretion

TABLE 9–6 (Continued)

Distal tubule (distal convoluted tubule and connecting tubule)

- Reabsorbs approximately 8% of the filtered Ca^{2+} load

- Major regulatory site of Ca^{2+} excretion by PTH

- Ca^{2+} transport is entirely active

- Transport is stimulated by PTH, alkalosis, and thiazide diuretics

- Transport is inhibited by acidosis and hypophosphatemia

Abbreviations: ECF, extracellular fluid; ROMK, renal outer medullary potassium; PTH, parathyroid hormone

HYPERCALCEMIA

TABLE 9–7: Etiologies of Hypercalcemia
Increased bone resorption
Hyperparathyroidism (primary and secondary)
Malignancy
Thyrotoxicosis
Immobilization
Paget's disease
Addison's disease
Lithium administration
Vitamin A intoxication
Familial hypocalciuric hypercalcemia
Increased GI absorption
Increased Ca^{2+} intake
• Milk-alkali syndrome
• CKD and ESRD (in patients given excessive Ca^{2+} and vitamin D supplementation)
Increased vitamin D concentration
• Vitamin D intoxication
• Granulomatous disease
Decreased renal excretion
Thiazide diuretics
Abbreviations: GI, gastrointestinal; CKD, chronic kidney disease; ESRD, end-stage renal disease

TABLE 9–8: Hypercalcemia—Increased GI Ca^{2+} Absorption

Milk-Alkali Syndrome

Pathophysiology

Results from excessive Ca^{2+} and bicarbonate intake or its equivalent

Alkalosis stimulates Ca^{2+} reabsorption in the distal tubule of kidney

Suppression of PTH secretion by hypercalcemia further increases proximal tubular bicarbonate reabsorption

Common causes

Most common cause of the milk-alkali syndrome in the past was milk and sodium bicarbonate ingestion for therapy of peptic ulcer disease

Today the most common clinical setting is an elderly woman treated with calcium carbonate and vitamin D for osteoporosis

Bulemics taking supplemental Ca^{2+} or a high Ca^{2+} diet are also at high risk

Presentation

Classic triad—hypercalcemia, metabolic alkalosis, and elevated BUN and creatinine concentrations

PTH concentrations are often very low

Beware of rebound hypocalcemia as a result of sustained PTH suppression from hypercalcemia; for this reason bisphosphonates should be used with caution in these patients; they should be reserved for those with severe hypocalcemia that are resistant to conventional therapy

(continued)

TABLE 9–8 (Continued)
Vitamin D Intoxication
Pathophysiology
Calcitriol stimulates Ca^{2+} absorption in small intestine, however, bone Ca^{2+} release may also play an important role
Common causes
A recent outbreak was reported as the result of over fortification of milk from a home delivery dairy
Other milk-associated outbreaks resulted from inadvertent calcitriol addition to milk
Granulomatous Disease
Pathophysiology
Macrophages express 1-α-hydroxylase when activated and convert calcidiol to calcitriol
Common causes
Sarcoidosis, mycobacterium tuberculosis, and mycobacterium avium in patients with HIV infection
Lymphomas can produce hypercalcemia via the same mechanism
Presentation
Hypercalcemia may be the initial manifestation of extrapulmonary sarcoid; this more commonly results in hypercalciuria than hypercalcemia
Abbreviations: GI, gastrointestinal; PTH, parathyroid hormone; BUN, blood urea nitrogen concentration; HIV, human immunodeficiency virus

TABLE 9–9: Hypercalcemia—Increased Bone Ca^{2+} Resorption (Hyperparathyroidism—Primary)

Ca^{2+} resorption from bone is the most common pathophysiologic mechanism leading to hypercalcemia

The two most common causes of hypercalcemia are primary hyperparathyroidism and malignancy

Primary Hyperparathyroidism

Pathophysiology

Hypercalcemia is the combined result of increased bone Ca^{2+} resorption, increased intestinal Ca^{2+} absorption, and increased Ca^{2+} reabsorption in kidney

Common causes

Ninety percent of patients have solitary adenomas

Of the remaining, as many as 10% have diffuse hyperplasia and some of these have the inherited familial syndrome MEN discussed further below

Multiple adenomas can occur and parathyroid carcinoma is very rare (< 1%)

Presentation

Occurs in as many as 1 per 10,000 people in the general population

Patients present most commonly between the ages of 40 and 60

Women are affected two to three times more often than men

The majority of patients are postmenopausal women

Hypercalcemia is mild (generally less than 11.0 mg/dL), and often identified on routine laboratory testing in the asymptomatic patient

Abbreviation: MEN, multiple endocrine neoplasia

TABLE 9–10: Hypercalcemia—Increased Bone Ca^{2+} Resorption (Hyperparathyroidism—Secondary)

Pathophysiology

Increased parathyroid gland mass

Nodular areas of the parathyroid gland have decreased expression of the Ca^{2+}-sensing and vitamin D receptors

Common causes

Post-renal transplant

Excess Ca^{2+} and/or vitamin D supplementation in patients with chronic kidney disease or end-stage renal disease

Presentation

In the renal transplant patient although renal function improves, PTH concentration is still elevated as a result of increased parathyroid gland mass; hypercalcemia generally does not persist more than a year

In the patient with chronic kidney disease or end-stage renal disease, hypercalcemia occurs primarily in patients with low turnover bone disease (adynamic bone disease) given supplemental Ca^{2+} and/or vitamin D

Abbreviation: PTH, parathyroid hormone

TABLE 9–11: Hypercalcemia—Increased Bone Ca^{2+} Resorption (Hyperparathyroidism—MEN Syndromes)

Pathophysiology

Menin is a tumor suppressor expressed in the nucleus that binds to JunD

RET is a tyrosine kinase; in developing tissues including neural crest, kidney, and ureter RET is a receptor for growth and differentiation

Common causes

MEN type I—the result of menin gene mutations

MEN type II—caused by mutations in the RET protooncogene

Presentation

Estimated prevalence of 1 per 50,000

MEN type I is associated with pituitary adenomas and islet cell tumors; primary hyperparathyroidism is the initial manifestation occurring in general by age 40–50

MEN type II is associated with medullary carcinoma of the thyroid and pheochromocytoma; it is subdivided into MEN IIa that is associated with parathyroid hyperplasia and type IIb that is not

Abbreviation: MEN, multiple endocrine neoplasia

TABLE 9–12: Hypercalcemia—Increased Bone Ca^{2+} Resorption (Malignancy—PTHrP Related)

Breast cancer, squamous cell lung cancer, multiple myeloma, and renal cell carcinoma are the most common malignancies associated with hypercalcemia
Pathophysiology
Seven of the first 13 amino acids of PTHrP are identical to PTH, and as a result PTHrP binds to the PTH receptor and has similar biologic activity to PTH
PTHrP may be the fetal PTH; PTH is not secreted by parathyroid gland in utero and does not cross the placenta
Common causes
A large variety of tumors can produce PTHrP; a partial list includes squamous cell cancers of the head, neck and lung, breast cancer, pancreatic cancer, transitional cell carcinomas, and germ cell tumors
Presentation
Typically presents with severe hypercalcemia (Ca^{2+} concentration >14 mg/dL)
At the time of initial presentation the cancer is usually easily identified
Humor hypercalcemia of malignancy carries a poor prognosis with a median survival of only 3 months
Diagnosis
PTH concentration is low
An assay for PTHrP is commercially available; PTHrP is immunologically distinct from PTH and as a result is not detected by PTH assays
Abbreviations: PTH, parathyroid hormone; PTHrP, parathyroid hormone-related protein

TABLE 9–13: Hypercalcemia—Increased Bone Ca^{2+} Resorption (Malignancy—Other Causes)

Multiple Myeloma

Pathophysiology

Ca^{2+} release from bone results from cytokine action (IL-6, IL-1, TNF-β, MIP-1-α, and MIP-1-β)

Myeloma cells also disturb the ratio of osteoprotegerin and its ligand NF-kappa B ligand (RANKL), which play a critical role in bone remodeling and the regulation of osteoclast and osteoblast activity

By decreasing expression and increasing degradation of osteoprotegerin and increasing RANKL expression in their local environment myeloma cells tip the balance in favor of bone resorption

Presentation

One-third of patients develop hypercalcemia

Patients present with anemia, hypercalcemia, and localized osteolytic lesions

Lytic bone lesions are characterized by increased osteoblast resorption without new bone formation; this is in contradistinction to bone metastases with breast and prostate cancer where areas of lysis are surrounded by new bone formation

Radionuclide bone scans will show uptake at sites of metastasis and not at sites of bone involvement with multiple myeloma

Diagnosis

Combination of SPEP, UPEP 24-h urine for IFE, and bone marrow aspirate and biopsy

(continued)

TABLE 9–13 (Continued)
Osteolytic Metastases
Osteolytic metastases produce a variety of cytokines resulting in bone Ca^{2+} release
TNF and interleukin-1 (IL-1) stimulate the differentiation of osteoclast precursors into osteoclasts
IL-6 stimulates osteoclast production
Calcitriol Production
Lymphomas can produce calcitriol; the source of activated vitamin D production may be from macrophages surrounding the tumor rather than the malignant lymphocytes themselves
Abbreviations: PTH, parathyroid hormone; SPEP, serum protein electrophoresis; UPEP, urine protein electrophoresis; IFE, immunofixation electrophoresis; TNF, tumor necrosis factor

TABLE 9–14: Hypercalcemia—FHH

FHH is important because it can be misdiagnosed as primary hyperparathyroidism and result in unnecessary parathyroid surgery

Pathophysiology

Autosomal dominant inheritance

Due to a mutation in the Ca^{2+}-sensing receptor that results in a receptor with decreased Ca^{2+} affinity

Elevated Ca^{2+} concentrations are required to suppress PTH

Presentation

Hypercalcemia at a young age

Decreased urinary Ca^{2+} excretion

High normal or slightly elevated PTH concentration

Signs and symptoms of hypercalcemia are often absent

Hypercalcemia is mild (generally less than 11.0 mg/dL), and often identified on routine laboratory testing in the asymptomatic patient

Patients with FHH often do not have clinical sequelae of excessive PTH activity such as hyperparathyroid bone disease or mental status changes

Diagnosis

Careful family history looking for hypercalcemia in family members

There should be a lack of previous normal serum Ca^{2+} measurements

Urinary calcium excretion is low

(continued)

TABLE 9–14 (Continued)

Caution

Some authors advocate using the FE of Ca^{2+} to distinguish FHH from primary hyperparathyroidism with values below 1% suggestive of FHH; it should be recognized, however, that is a subgroup of patients with primary hyperparathyroidism that have a fractional excretion of Ca^{2+} below 1%

Abbreviations: FHH, familial hypocalciuric hypercalcemia; PTH, parathyroid hormone; FE, fractional excretion

TABLE 9–15: Hypercalcemia—Other Causes

Increased bone Ca^{2+} resorption

- Hyperthyroidism

  - Mild hypercalcemia occurs in 5–10%

  - There may also be an increased incidence of parathyroid adenomas

- Immobilization

  - Hypercalcemia more common in children, usually causes hypercalciuria in adults

- Paget's disease

  - Hypercalcemia more common in children, usually causes hypercalciuria in adults

- Lithium administration

  - Lithium interferes with Ca^{2+} sensing by the Ca^{2+}-sensing receptor

  - Generally results in only mild hypercalcemia that generally resolves with drug discontinuation

- Pheochromocytoma

  - May produce hypercalcemia via its association with MEN IIa or by PTHrP production

  - Catecholamines are also known to increase bone resorption

- Addison's disease

Increased renal Ca^{2+} reabsorption

- Thiazide diuretics

  - Increase distal nephron Ca^{2+} reabsorption

  - Most reported cases were associated with parathyroid adenomas

Abbreviations: MEN, multiple endocrine neoplasia; PTHrP, parathyroid hormone-related protein

TABLE 9–16: Signs and Symptoms

The extent of clinical signs and symptoms are determined by the severity and rate of rise of the Ca^{2+} concentration

Patients with primary hyperparathyroidism present with mild asymptomatic hypercalcemia incidentally discovered on routine laboratory examination; malignancy presents often with severe, symptomatic hypercalcemia

Neurologic

Central nervous system symptoms range from confusion to stupor and coma

Seizures can occur as a result of severe vasoconstriction and transient high intensity signals have been documented by MRI that resolve with return of serum Ca^{2+} to the normal range

Focal neurologic symptoms mimicking a transient ischemic attack although rare are described

Gastrointestinal

Decreased gastrointestinal motility results in nausea and vomiting

Hypercalcemia-induced pancreatitis can cause epigastric pain

Systemic

ECF volume depletion—hypercalcemia decreases expression of water channels resulting in polyuria

Decreased renal function from prerenal azotemia (ECF volume contraction)

Predisposes to digitalis toxicity

Abbreviations: MRI, magnetic resonance imaging; ECF, extracellular fluid

TABLE 9–17: Diagnosis

Primary hyperparathyroidism and malignancy are by far the most frequent causes making up more than 90% of all cases

Primary hyperparathyroidism is generally the cause in asymptomatic outpatients with a serum Ca^{2+} concentration below 11 mg/dL

Malignancy is the most common cause in symptomatic patients with serum Ca^{2+} concentration above 14 mg/dL

Factors favoring the diagnosis of primary hyperparathyroidism include a prolonged history, development in a postmenopausal woman, a normal physical examination, and evidence of MEN

Initial evaluation

Careful history and physical examination

Of patients with primary hyperparathyroidism about 20% have signs and symptoms of disease such as kidney stones, neuromuscular weakness, decreased ability to concentrate, depression, or bone disease

One should inquire carefully about Ca^{2+} supplement use, antacids, and vitamin preparations

A recent chest radiograph is essential to exclude lung cancers and granulomatous diseases

In patients with primary hyperparathyroidism skeletal radiographs are rarely positive in the present era; bone densitometry, however, is commonly abnormal; since primary hyperparathyroidism involves cortical more than cancellous bone, bone density is reduced to the greatest degree in distal radius; areas where cancellous bone predominates such as the spine and hip show less of a decrease

Abbreviation: MEN, multiple endocrine neoplasia

TABLE 9–18: Diagnosis (Clinical Laboratory)

Laboratory examination

Initial laboratory studies include electrolytes, BUN, creatinine, phosphorus, serum and urine protein electrophoresis, and a 24-h urine collection for Ca^{2+} and creatinine; if hyperthyroidism is suspected, thyroid function tests are obtained

A ratio of serum Cl^- to serum phosphorus concentrations of greater than 33:1 is suggestive of primary hyperparathyroidism; this results from decreased proximal tubular phosphate reabsorption induced by PTH

Laboratory hallmarks of milk-alkali syndrome are a low serum Cl^-, high serum bicarbonate, and elevated serum BUN and creatinine concentrations

A monoclonal gammopathy on serum or urine protein electrophoresis suggests multiple myeloma; if the diagnosis of multiple myeloma is suspected on clinical grounds, it is important to perform IFE on both blood and a 24-h urine sample in order to exclude the diagnosis

In primary hyperparathyroidism and humoral hypercalcemia of malignancy serum phosphorus concentration is often low

In hypercalcemia resulting from milk-alkali syndrome, thiazide diuretics, and FHH 24-h urinary Ca^{2+} excretion will be low

Evaluation of serum PTH and PTHrP concentrations

Primary hyperparathyroidism is the most common cause of an elevated PTH; PTH concentration is generally 1.5–2.0 times the upper limit of normal

TABLE 9–18 (Continued)

Some patients may have mildly elevated Ca^{2+} with a PTH concentration that is in the upper range of normal (inappropriately elevated); others may have a serum Ca^{2+} concentration in the upper quartile of the normal range and a slightly elevated PTH concentration; both of these subgroups of patients were demonstrated to have parathyroid adenomas

An elevated PTH concentration may be seen rarely with lithium and FHH; if the patient is on lithium and it can be safely discontinued PTH concentration should be remeasured in 1–3 months; in all other etiologies PTH is suppressed

PTHrP is immunologically distinct from PTH and specific assays are commercially available; C-terminal fragment PTHrP assays may be increased in pregnancy and in patients with chronic kidney disease

Evaluation of serum calcidiol and calcitriol concentrations

If malignancy is not obvious and PTH concentration is suppressed, one needs to rule out vitamin D intoxication or granulomatous diseases by measuring calcidiol and calcitriol concentrations

Vitamin D or calcidiol ingestion will result in an increased calcidiol concentration and often mild to moderately elevated calcitriol concentration

Elevated calcitriol concentration is observed with calcitriol ingestion and in those diseases where stimulation of 1-α-hydroxylase occurs including granulomatous diseases, lymphoma, and primary hyperparathyroidism

Abbreviations: BUN, blood urea nitrogen; IFE, immunofixation electrophoresis; FHH, familial hypocalciuric hypercalcemia; PTH, parathyroid hormone; PTHrP, parathyroid hormone-related protein

TABLE 9–19: Treatment (Medical—General Principles)

Treatment of hypercalcemia will depend on the degree of serum Ca^{2+} concentration elevation and is directed at increasing renal excretion, blocking bone resorption, and reducing intestinal absorption

Volume expansion and loop diuretics alone may be sufficient in the patient with mild-to-moderate hypercalcemia ($\leq$12.5 mg/dL)

When hypercalcemia is moderate or severe bone Ca^{2+} resorption must be inhibited

Agents that decrease intestinal Ca^{2+} absorption are generally reserved for outpatients with mild hypercalcemia

Increasing Renal Excretion

Expansion of ECF volume—the hypercalcemic patient is almost always volume contracted

- Hypercalcemia causes arteriolar vasoconstriction and reduces renal blood flow

- Ca^{2+} acts directly in the thick ascending limb of Henle to decrease Na^+ reabsorption and promotes natriuresis

- Hypercalcemia also antagonizes antidiuretic hormone effects in collecting duct

- Volume contraction increases proximal Na^+ and Ca^{2+} reabsorption and further increases serum Ca^{2+} concentration

Loop diuretics

- Dissipate the lumen-positive voltage and reduce Ca^{2+} reabsorption in the thick ascending limb of the loop of Henle

TABLE 9–19 (Continued)

- The goal is to maintain urine flow rate at 200–250 mL/h

- With chronic kidney disease higher doses of loop diuretics are required

Hemodialysis

- If GFR is low and hypercalcemia severe ($\geq$ 17 mg/dL), hemodialysis may be indicated

- Hemodialysis is also helpful in patients with neurologic impairment or in those with concomitant congestive heart failure

Abbreviations: ECF, extracellular fluid; GFR, glomerular filtration rate

TABLE 9–20: Treatment (Medical—Blocking Bone Resorption-I)

Calcitonin

- Used in the short-term because of its rapid onset (within a few hours)

- Usual dose is 4 IU/kg subcutaneously every 12 h

- It not only inhibits bone resorption but also increases renal Ca^{2+} excretion

- Its effect is not large and serum Ca^{2+} concentration is reduced by only 1–2 mg/dL

- Tachyphylaxis develops with repeated use

- Should be used with another agent that decreases bone resorption

Bisphosphonates

- The drug of choice to inhibit bone resorption

- Effects are additive with calcitonin

- Bisphosphonates are concentrated in bone where they interfere with osteoclast formation, recruitment, activation, and function

- They have a long duration of action (weeks) but their disadvantage is that they have a slow onset (48–72 h)

- Pamidronate is frequently used; 60 or 90 mg is given intravenously over 2–4 h; the dose varies depending on the degree of hypercalcemia (60 mg when Ca^{2+} concentration < 13.5 mg/dL, 90 mg when Ca^{2+} concentration > 13.5 mg/dL); serum Ca^{2+} concentration slowly falls over days and normalizes within 7 days; a single dose lasts 7–14 days

TABLE 9–20 (Continued)

- Zolendronic acid is another bisphosphonate that is commonly used because it can be given over short intervals (4 mg over 15 min or longer); its effect may persist longer than pamidronate and it is administered every 3–4 weeks. The manufacturer recommends dosage reduction for decreases in creatinine clearance: > 60 ml/min- 4mg; 50–60 ml/min- 3.5 mg; 40–49 ml/min- 3.3 mg; 30–39 ml/min- 3.0mg; < 30 ml/min- insufficient data. Serum creatinine concentration should be followed closely during zolendronic acid administration. The manufacturer also states that the drug should be discontinued if serum creatinine concentration increases ≥ 0.5 mg/dL in patients with normal baseline levels or if it increases ≥ 1.0 mg/dL in patients with serum creatinine concentrations ≥ 1.4 mg/dL

- Renal toxicities of bisphosphonates include focal glomerulosclerosis with pamidronate and acute kidney injury with zolendronate and pamidronate

- Bisphosphonates particulary when used in the long-term treatment of malignancies complicated by hypercalcemia have been associated with osteonecrosis of the jaw

TABLE 9–21: Treatment (Medical—Blocking Bone Resorption-II)

Mithramycin—rarely used

- Cannot be used in patients with severe liver, kidney, or bone marrow disease

- Onset of action is 12 h with a peak effect at 48 h

- Due to its severe side-effect profile (hepatotoxicity, proteinuria, thrombocytopenia, and GI upset) it is rarely used

- The dose is 25 μg/kg intravenously over 4 h daily for 3–4 days

- In one study hepatotoxicity was noted in 26% of patients, nausea and vomiting in 23%, as well as bleeding tendencies due to abnormalities in several coagulation factors and platelet dysfunction

Gallium nitrate—rarely used

- Accumulates in metabolically active regions of bone

- Reduces bone resorption by inhibiting the H^+ATPase in the ruffled membrane of osteoclasts and blocking osteoclast acid secretion

- Used to treat hypercalcemia of malignancy

- One hundred to two hundred mg/m^2 is given as a continuous infusion for 5 consecutive days

- Contraindicated if serum creatinine concentration is above 2.5 mg/dL

Abbreviations: GI, gastrointestinal; ATP, adenosine triphosphate

TABLE 9–22: Treatment (Medical—Reducing Intestinal Absorption)

Corticosteroids

- Used successfully in patients with vitamin D overdose, granulomatous diseases, and some cancers (lymphomas and multiple myeloma); the usual dose of prednisone is 20–40 mg/day

Ketoconazole and hydroxychloroquine

- Ketoconazole reduces calcitriol concentration by approximately 75% via inhibition of 1-α-hydroxylase

  - Dose range 200–800 mg/day, usually requires higher doses

  - Many potential drug interactions

- Hydroxychloroquine was used in patients with hypercalcemia caused by sarcoidosis and works via a similar mechanism

  - Dose range 200–400 mg/day

  - Patient should be carefully monitored for ocular toxicity

Oral phosphorus

- Contraindicated in patients with an elevated serum phosphorus concentration or renal dysfunction

- Usual dose 250–500 mg four times a day

- Often poorly tolerated at higher doses (diarrhea)

- Reduces Ca^{2+} concentration only slightly (1 mg/dL)

TABLE 9–23: Treatment (Surgical)

Whether to surgically remove a solitary parathyroid adenoma remains controversial

Criteria for surgical removal

- Serum Ca^{2+} concentration more than 1 mg/dL above the upper limit of normal

- An episode of acute symptomatic hypercalcemia

- Overt bone disease-cortical bone mineral density more than two standard deviations below age, sex, and race adjusted means

- Reduced renal function (more than 30%)

- A history of nephrolithiasis or nephrocalcinosis

- Urinary Ca^{2+} excretion that exceeds 400 mg/day

- Age less than 50 years

Other considerations

- At least half of affected patients will meet the above criteria

- In approximately 75% of patients who do not elect surgery, average serum Ca^{2+} and PTH concentrations generally do not change

- In the remaining 25% signs and symptoms worsen with increasing hypercalcemia, hypercalciuria, and decreasing bone mineral density

- Patients below the age of 50 and those with nephrolithiasis are at higher risk of progression

- If surgery is not performed it is recommended that serum Ca^{2+} concentration be monitored every 6 months and serum creatinine concentration and bone mineral density measured yearly

TABLE 9–23 (Continued)

Surgical results

- In patients whose surgery is successful the rate of kidney stone formation declines

- Over the next several years bone density often increases in hip and back but not in the distal third of the radius

- Patients treated medically with bisphosphonates can have some increase in vertebral bone density but serum PTH concentrations remain elevated

- Ca^{2+}-sensing receptor agonists can normalize serum Ca^{2+} concentration but in studies of up to 3 years duration bone density does not increase

Abbreviation: PTH, parathyroid hormone

TABLE 9–24: Minimally Invasive Parathyroid Surgery

As minimally invasive parathyroid surgery becomes more accepted surgical criteria will be broadened

The technique

- With minimally invasive surgery adenomas are first localized with a sestamibi scan and/or ultrasound preoperatively and parathyroidectomy is performed under local anesthesia

- PTH assays are performed in the operating room

- Given PTH's short half-life (4 min), after the adenoma is removed PTH concentration is remeasured to verify that surgery was successful. The PTH level should decrease > 50% from the preincision intraoperative value 10 min after adenoma removal

- If PTH concentration does not decline, the patient is placed under general anesthesia and more extensive neck exploration is performed looking for a second adenoma

- Up to 5% of patients may have a previously undetected second adenoma

Abbreviation: PTH, parathyroid hormone

HYPOCALCEMIA

TABLE 9–25: Pathophysiologic Mechanisms
Hypocalcemia results from decreased intestinal Ca^{2+} absorption or decreased bone resorption
Since there is a large Ca^{2+} reservoir in bone sustained hypocalcemia can only occur if there is an abnormality of PTH or calcitriol effect in bone
True hypocalcemia results only when the ionized Ca^{2+} fraction is decreased (about half of total serum Ca^{2+} concentration)
Normal range for ionized Ca^{2+} concentration is 4.2–5.0 mg/dL or 1.05–1.25 mmol/L
Abbreviation: PTH, parathyroid hormone

TABLE 9–26: Etiologies of Hypocalcemia

True hypocalcemia is the result of either decreased PTH or vitamin D concentration or end-organ resistance; less commonly, hypocalcemia results from either extravascular Ca^{2+} deposition or intravascular Ca^{2+} binding

Decreased PTH action or effect

Hypomagnesemia

Decreased PTH secretion

- Postsurgical

- Polyglandular autoimmune syndrome type I

- Familial hypocalcemia

- Infiltrative disorders

End-organ resistance to PTH

- Pseudohypoparathyroidism (type I and II)

Defects in vitamin D metabolism

Nutritional

Malabsorption

Drugs

Liver disease

Renal disease

Vitamin D-dependent rickets

Ca^{2+} shift out of the ECF

Acute pancreatitis

Hungry bone syndrome

Tumor lysis syndrome

TABLE 9–26 (Continued)
Intravascular Ca^{2+} binding
Foscarnet use (pyrophosphate analogue)
Massive transfusion (citrate)—often in the presence of hepatic or renal dysfunction
Miscellaneous
Osteoblastic metastases
Toxic shock syndrome
Sepsis
Pseudohypocalcemia
Abbreviations: PTH, parathyroid hormone; ECF, extracellular fluid

TABLE 9–27: Hypocalcemia—Secondary to Disorders of Decreased PTH Synthesis or Release—Hypomagnesemia

Hypoparathyroidism is caused by several acquired and inherited disorders resulting from decreased PTH synthesis or release, or resistance to PTH action
Hypomagnesemia
Pathophysiology
Hypomagnesemia decreases PTH secretion, as well as results in end-organ resistance to PTH
End-organ resistance begins to occur at serum Mg^{2+} concentration ≤1.0 mg/dL
More severe hypomagnesemia (serum Mg^{2+} concentration ≤ 0.5 mg/dL) is required to decrease PTH secretion
Presentation
The most common etiology of decreased PTH secretion and/or effect is severe hypomagnesemia
Patients with hypocalcemia secondary to hypomagnesemia will not respond to Ca^{2+} or vitamin D replacement until the Mg^{2+} deficit is replaced
It often takes several days after the Mg^{2+} deficit is corrected for serum Ca^{2+} concentration to return to normal
Diagnosis
Measurement of serum magnesium concentration
High index of suspicion
Abbreviation: PTH, parathyroid hormone

TABLE 9–28: Hypocalcemia—Secondary to Disorders of Decreased PTH Synthesis or Release-Other Causes

Polyglandular autoimmune syndrome type I

Pathophysiology

Mutations in the AIRE gene (autoimmune regulator), which is a transcription factor, cause the disease

Up to half of patients have antibodies directed against the Ca^{2+}-sensing receptor

Presentation

The most common cause of idiopathic hypoparathyroidism

Chronic mucocutaneous candidiasis and primary adrenal insufficiency are also part of this disease

Mucocutaneous candidiasis presents in early childhood and involves skin and mucous membranes without systemic spread; this is subsequently followed by hypoparathyroidism after several years

Adrenal insufficiency generally develops last with an onset in adolescence

Affected patients are at risk for developing other autoimmune disorders including pernicious anemia, vitiligo, hypothyroidism, hepatitis, and type I diabetes mellitus

Diagnosis

PTH concentration is low

Serum Ca^{2+} concentration is low in the presence of hyperphosphatemia

(continued)

TABLE 9–28 (Continued)

Familial hypocalcemia

- Autosomal dominant activating mutations in the Ca^{2+}-sensing receptor result in a receptor that is more sensitive to ECF ionized Ca^{2+} concentration

- Two patients were described with autoantibodies that activate the Ca^{2+}-sensing receptor; one patient had Graves's disease and the other Addison's disease

Radical neck or previous parathyroid surgery

Post parathyroid adenoma removal—usually transient

Infiltrative disorders

- Hemochromatosis

- Wilson's disease

HIV infection

Post-thyroid surgery

- Can be either transient (11.9%) or permanent (0.9%)

- Patients undergoing central lymph node dissection for thyroid cancer are at high risk

- Hypocalcemia or hypophosphatemia that persists for 1 week despite Ca^{2+} replacement are risk factors for permanent hypoparathyroidism

Abbreviations: PTH, parathyroid hormone; ECF, extracellular fluid

TABLE 9–29: Hypocalcemia—Secondary to Disorders of End-Organ Resistance to PTH

Hypomagnesemia (see Table 9–27)

Pseudohypoparathyroidism types I and II

- Rare genetic disorders—usually autosomal dominant inheritance

- Associated with short stature, obesity, round facies, subcutaneous ossifications, and brachydactyly

- Pseudohypoparathyroidism is subdivided based on whether nephrogenous cAMP increases in response to PTH administration (Ellsworth-Howard test)

- In type II there is a normal response and in type I there is a decreased response

- In type I the mutation arises in the $Gs\alpha_1$-protein of the adenylate cyclase complex; parathyroid hormone binds to its receptor but cannot activate adenylate cyclase

- The defect in type II is due to resistance to the intracellular effects of cyclic AMP and the mutation has yet to be identified; some patients with type II disease will respond to theophylline

- Serum Ca^{2+} concentration is low, serum phosphorus concentration high, and PTH concentration is elevated

Abbreviations: cAMP, cyclic AMP; PTH, parathyroid hormone; AMP, adenosine monophosphate

TABLE 9–30: Hypocalcemia—Disorders Secondary to Defects in Vitamin D Metabolism

Disorders of vitamin D metabolism are important causes of hypocalcemia; a wide variety of disorders can interfere with this complex pathway

Decreased vitamin D intake

- Despite the fact that milk is supplemented with vitamin D in the U.S.; one study of noninstitutionalized adults showed that 9% had low 25(OH) vitamin D_3 concentration

- Patients who are poorly nourished with little sunlight exposure (i.e.; the institutionalized elderly) are at risk

- Postmenopausal women and adolescents are also at increased risk

GI malabsorption

- Vitamin D is a fat-soluble vitamin

Drugs

- Anticonvulsant drugs induce the cytochrome P450 system and increase metabolism of vitamin D; in addition, they inhibit bone resorption, impair GI Ca^{2+} absorption, and cause resistance to PTH action

Liver disease

- An important step in vitamin D metabolism involves 25-hydroxylation in liver

Chronic kidney disease

- Impairs 1-α-hydroxylation—the final step in the formation of calcitriol

TABLE 9–30 (Continued)

Vitamin D-dependent rickets

- Type I is caused by impaired 1-α-hydroxylation of calcidiol to calcitriol; since end-organ response is intact type I patients respond to calcitriol

- Type II disease is caused by inactivating mutations in the vitamin D receptor and results in end-organ resistance to calcitriol; serum calcitriol concentration is elevated and these patients respond poorly to supplemental calcitriol

Abbreviations: PTH, parathyroid hormone; GI, gastrointestinal

TABLE 9–31: Hypocalcemia—Other Causes

Ca^{2+} shift out of the ECF

- Acute pancreatitis
  - Ca^{2+} binding to free fatty acids and deposition in soft tissues
  - Inadequate parathyroid response
- Hungry bone syndrome
- Tumor lysis syndrome
  - Hyperphosphatemia reduces Ca^{2+} efflux from bone
  - Calcium phosphate complex deposition in soft tissues

Intravascular Ca^{2+} binding

- Foscarnet use
  - Pyrophosphate analogue
- Massive transfusion (citrate)
  - Often in the presence of hepatic or renal dysfunction

Miscellaneous

- Osteoblastic metastases
- Toxic shock syndrome
- Sepsis
  - Ionized hypocalcemia is common in patients in the ICU occurring in up to one-third to two-thirds and many of these are septic
  - Hypocalcemia is an independent predictor of increased mortality in the ICU; the mechanism of hypocalcemia in sepsis is unknown

TABLE 9–31 (Continued)

- Postulated mechanisms include a decrease in PTH concentration, decreased calcitriol concentration, and peripheral resistance to PTH action

Pseudohypocalcemia

- Some preparations of Gadolinium, used as a contrast agent in magnetic resonance imaging, interfere with some assays used to measure serum Ca^{2+} concentration

- The effect is short lived in patients with normal renal function (3–6 h) but can result in very low spurious Ca^{2+} determinations (decreases of 3 mg/dL or more); the patients, as expected, exhibit no symptoms. In patients with severe renal dysfunction hypocalcemia may persist for as long as 4 days

Abbreviations: ECF, extracellular fluid; ICU, intensive care unit; PTH, parathyroid hormone

TABLE 9–32: Signs and Symptoms

The degree of hypocalcemia and rate of decline of serum Ca^{2+} concentration determine whether hypocalcemic symptoms occur

The point at which symptoms occur depends on multiple factors including pH, and whether other electrolyte abnormalities are present (hypomagnesemia and hypokalemia)

Neuromuscular

Altered mental status changes, irritability, and seizures

Circumoral and distal extremity paresthesias

Carpopedal spasm

Physical examination

Hypotension and bradycardia

Laryngospasm

Chvostek's sign

- Brought out by gently tapping just below the zygomatic arch over the facial nerve with the mouth slightly open

- A positive sign, which is a facial twitch, is occasionally observed in normal patients

Trousseau's sign

- A blood pressure cuff is inflated to 20 mmHg above systolic pressure for 3 min

- A positive sign is flexion of the wrist, metacarpophalyngeal joints, and thumb with hyperextension of the fingers

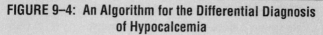

FIGURE 9–4: An Algorithm for the Differential Diagnosis of Hypocalcemia

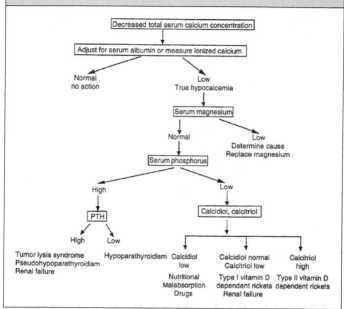

TABLE 9–33: Approach to the Patient with a Low Total Serum Ca^{2+} Concentration

Common causes are hypomagnesemia (most common), chronic kidney disease, and postparathyroid surgery

Step 1 Determine whether the ionized Ca^{2+} fraction is reduced (does the patient have true hypocalcemia)

- Compare the total serum Ca^{2+} concentration to the serum albumin concentration

- As a general rule of thumb for every 1 g/dL decrease in serum albumin concentration from its normal value (4 g/dL), one can expect a 0.8 mg/dL decrement in total serum Ca^{2+} concentration; for every 1 g/dL fall in serum albumin concentration, 0.8 mg/dL must be added to the total serum Ca^{2+} concentration to correct it for the degree of hypoalbuminemia

- Prediction of ionized Ca^{2+} from albumin-corrected total Ca^{2+} should be done with caution; this correction may be unreliable in certain patient populations such as the critically ill trauma patient

- Ca^{2+} binding to albumin is also affected by pH; as pH decreases ionized Ca^{2+} will increase and vice versa; this effect is fairly minor and ionized serum Ca^{2+} concentration will only increase 0.2 mg/dL for each 0.1 decrease in pH

- If clinical suspicion of true hypocalcemia is high then ionized Ca^{2+} concentration should be measured directly

- After the presence of true hypocalcemia is established, blood is sent for BUN, creatinine, Mg^{2+}, and phosphorus concentrations

Step 2 Evaluate the serum Mg^{2+} concentration

- The most common cause of hypocalcemia is hypomagnesemia

- Hypocalcemia will not correct before Mg^{2+} deficits are replenished

TABLE 9–33 (Continued)

Step 3 Examine the serum phosphorus concentration

- Hyperphosphatemia

  - Elevated BUN and creatinine concentrations suggest chronic kidney disease

  - If kidney function is normal hyperphosphatemia suggests hypoparathyroidism or pseudohypoparathyroidism

  - These disorders can be differentiated by measuring PTH concentration

  - PTH concentration is low in primary hypoparathyroidism due to gland failure, whereas with end-organ resistance as in pseudohypoparathyroidism PTH concentration is elevated

  - Tumor lysis syndrome results in acute phosphorus release from cells that secondarily lowers serum Ca^{2+} concentration

- Hypophosphatemia

  - Disorders of vitamin D metabolism are characterized by hypophosphatemia

  - Hypocalcemia stimulates the parathyroid gland to secrete PTH that results in renal phosphate wasting; the FE of phosphorus will be high (> 5%)

  - These disorders are subdivided by measuring serum calcidiol and calcitriol concentrations

  - Calcidiol levels are low with malabsorption, liver disease, phenobarbital, nutritional deficiency, and nephrotic syndrome

  - Calcitriol levels are low with chronic kidney disease and increased in type II vitamin D-dependent rickets

Abbreviations: BUN, blood urea nitrogen; PTH, parathyroid hormone; FE, fractional excretion

TABLE 9–34: Treatment—Inpatients

Treatment will vary depending on the degree and cause of hypocalcemia

Life-threatening symptoms present—seizures, tetany, hypotension, or cardiac arrhythmias

- IV Ca^{2+} should be used initially in the symptomatic patient or the patient with severe hypocalcemia (total Ca^{2+} corrected for albumin $\leq$ 7.5 mg/dL); 100–300 mg is administered over 10–15 min

- A variety of IV preparations can be used including 10% Ca gluconate; (1) 10 mL ampules (94 mg of elemental Ca^{2+}); (2) 10% Ca gluceptate—5 mL ampule (90 mg elemental Ca^{2+}); and (3) CaCl—10 mL ampule (272 mg elemental Ca^{2+})

- After the first ampule is administered generally over several minutes, an infusion is then begun at 0.5–1.0 mg/kg/h; the infusion rate is subsequently adjusted based on serial serum Ca^{2+} determinations

The patient with severe hypocalcemia—without life-threatening symptoms

- If life-threatening symptoms are not present the administration of 15 mg/kg of elemental Ca^{2+} over 4–6 h can be expected to increase total serum Ca^{2+} concentration by 2–3 mg/dL

Mild hypocalcemia

- Hypocalcemia that is mild is corrected with oral Ca^{2+} supplementation (see Table 9–36)

- A vitamin D preparation may be added if the response to oral Ca^{2+} is insufficient

TABLE 9–34 (Continued)
Caution
• Mg^{2+} deficits must first be corrected or treatment will be ineffective
• In the patient who also has metabolic acidosis, hypocalcemia should be corrected first if possible; correction of acidosis before hypocalcemia will result in a further decrease in ionized Ca^{2+} concentration and exacerbate symptoms
• In the presence of severe hyperphosphatemia it is advisable to delay Ca^{2+} supplementation until serum phosphorus concentration is below 6 mg/dL; this may not always be possible and clinical judgment must be used
• Patients with hypocalcemia postparathyroidectomy require large doses of supplemental Ca^{2+}; in this setting the serum K^+ must be monitored carefully since for unclear reasons these patients are at increased risk of hyperkalemia
Abbreviation: IV, intravenous

TABLE 9–35: Oral Ca^{2+} Preparations		
Preparation	**Tablet (mg)**	**Elemental Ca^{2+}/ Tablet (mg)**
Ca^{2+} carbonate	500	200
Ca^{2+} citrate	950	200
Ca^{2+} lactate	650	85
Ca^{2+} gluconate	1000	90

TABLE 9–36: Oral Vitamin D Preparations			
Preparation	**Form of Vitamin D**	**Capsule Size**	**Dose**
Ergocalciferol	Vitamin D_2	50,000 IU/capsule	10,000–200,000 IU/day
Calcifediol	25 OH vitamin D_3	20, 50 µg/capsule	20–200 µg/day
Calcitriol	1,25$(OH)_2$ vitamin D_3	0.25, 0.5 µg/capsule	0.25 QOD to 2 µg/day
Abbreviation: QOD, every other day			

TABLE 9–37: Treatment—Outpatients

Ca^{2+} concentration should be maintained at a level where the patient is symptom free; this is generally at or just below the lower limit of normal

Oral Ca^{2+} supplements

- An elemental Ca^{2+} dose of 1–3 g/day is usually required; if higher doses are needed, a vitamin D preparation should be added

- Supplements should be taken between meals to ensure optimal absorption

- Calcium citrate is more bioavailable than calcium carbonate especially in patients with increased gastric pH

Vitamin D preparations

- Vitamin D supplements are often required if oral Ca^{2+} alone is ineffective

- Calcitriol is the most potent vitamin D preparation, has a rapid onset of action, a short duration of action, but is also the most expensive; a dose of 0.5–1.0 µg/day is often required

- As one moves from calcitriol to calcifediol, to ergocalciferol cost decreases; ergocalciferol requires 25 hydroxylation in the liver and 1 hydroxylation in kidney; calcifediol requires 1 hydroxylation in kidney; these agents are less efficacious in the presence of renal or hepatic disease

- As one moves from calcitriol to calcifediol, to ergocalciferol the duration of action increases, as a result the time to a rise in serum Ca^{2+} concentration increases, and the time for reversal of any toxic effects increases

(continued)

TABLE 9–37 (Continued)

Caution

- In hypoparathyroidism distal tubular Ca^{2+} reabsorption is decreased due to a lack of PTH; the increased filtered Ca^{2+} load resulting from Ca^{2+} and vitamin D replacement can lead to hypercalciuria, nephrolithiasis, and nephrocalcinosis

- Patients with hypoparathyroidism excrete more Ca^{2+} than normal for any given serum Ca^{2+} concentration; if urinary Ca^{2+} excretion exceeds 350 mg/day and serum Ca^{2+} concentration is acceptable, Na^+ intake should be restricted and if this is not effective a thiazide diuretic added in order to reduce urinary Ca^{2+} excretion

Abbreviation: PTH, parathyroid hormone

10
Disorders of Serum Phosphorus

REGULATION

TABLE 10–1: Phosphorus Homeostasis—Overview
Phosphorus circulates in the bloodstream in two forms, an organic fraction and an inorganic fraction; it is the inorganic fraction that is assayed in the clinical laboratory
The normal range is 2.5–4.5 mg/dL
Phosphorus fractions in blood
• Seventy-five percent of inorganic phosphorus is free in solution and exists as either divalent (HPO_4^{2-}) or monovalent ($H_2PO_4^-$) phosphate; the relative amounts of each ion depend on systemic pH; at pH 7.4, 80% is in the divalent form
• Fifteen percent is protein bound
• A small fraction of inorganic phosphorus is complexed with Ca^{2+} or Mg^{2+}
In normal individuals serum phosphorus concentration is at its lowest in the morning, gradually rises during the day and peaks shortly after midnight
• Diurnal variation in serum phosphorus concentration may be as much as 1 mg/dL
The largest reservoir of phosphorus in the body is in the skeleton (80%)
• The majority of the remainder is in skeletal muscle and viscera with only 1% in ECF
• Of the intracellular pool only a very small fraction is inorganic and can be used for the synthesis of high-energy phosphate-containing molecules (adenosine triphosphate)
Abbreviation: ECF, extracellular fluid

TABLE 10–2: Phosphorus Fluxes between ECF and Organ Systems
On average approximately 800–1400 mg of phosphorus is ingested daily
Of this total 640–1120 mg is absorbed primarily in the duodenum and jejunum
• The majority of phosphorus absorption in intestine is passive but there is a small active component regulated by vitamin D
In large intestine there is a component of unregulated secretion (100–200 mg/day) that can increase with diarrhea and contribute to hypophosphatemia
PTH and calcitriol are important regulators of phosphorus homeostasis via their actions in bone, intestine, and kidney
A newly described "phosphatonin" FGF-23 may play a role in normal phosphorus homeostasis
Abbreviations: ECF, extracellular fluid; PTH, paratyroid hormone; FGF, fibroblast growth factor

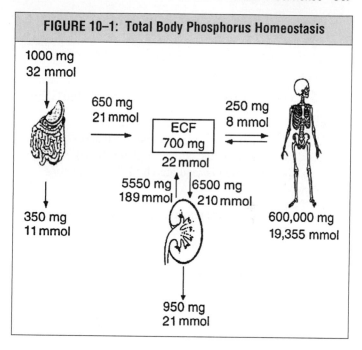

FIGURE 10–1: Total Body Phosphorus Homeostasis

1000 mg
32 mmol

650 mg
21 mmol

250 mg
8 mmol

ECF
700 mg
22 mmol

5550 mg
189 mmol

6500 mg
210 mmol

350 mg
11 mmol

600,000 mg
19,355 mmol

950 mg
21 mmol

TABLE 10–3: Renal Phosphorus Handling
Renal phosphate excretion is the prime regulator of serum phosphorus concentration
• The majority is reabsorbed in proximal tubule (80%) and this is the major regulatory site
• Phosphate enters the proximal tubular cell across the apical membrane via the Na^+-phosphate (NaPi) cotransporter, which is regulated by PTH and dietary phosphorus intake
• The kidney can reduce phosphorus excretion to very low levels in phosphorus depletion
Three types of Na-phosphate cotransporters are expressed in kidney (NaPi-I, -II, and -III)
• NaPi-II is further subdivided into three isoforms—a, b, and c
• NaPi-IIa is the major isoform in proximal tubule
Abbreviation: PTH, parathyroid hormone

TABLE 10–4: Na-Phosphate Cotransporter Isoforms			
Isoforms	Phosphate Transported (%)	Cellular Localization	Transport Mode
NaPi-I	15	Apical	Electrogenic
NaPi-II	84	Apical	
a			Electrogenic
b			Electrogenic
c			Electroneutral
NaPi-III	0.5	Basolateral	Electrogenic

TABLE 10–5: NaPi Regulation

Dietary phosphorus intake and PTH regulate NaPi-IIa

- NaPi-IIa is electrogenic and transports three Na^+ ions for each HPO_4^{2-} and is expressed in the apical membrane (urine side) of the proximal tubule

- Both PTH and high dietary phosphorus intake result in endocytic retrieval of NaPi-IIa from the brush border membrane to small endocytic vesicles

- Endocytic vesicles are shuttled to lysosomes by a microtubule-mediated process and degraded; there is little to no recycling

NaPi-IIb is expressed in the brush border of enterocytes; it lacks the dibasic amino acid motif (RK) at the C-terminus that is critical for endocytosis and is not regulated by PTH

- The primary upregulators of NaPi-IIb are a low phosphorus diet and calcitriol

- NaPi-IIb expression is also stimulated by estrogens and inhibited by glucocorticoids and epidermal growth factor

Abbreviations: NaPi, sodium phosphate; PTH, parathyroid hormone

TABLE 10–6: Phosphorus Regulation—PTH and Calcitriol

PTH and calcitriol exert effects in bone, kidney, and intestine

PTH maintains serum Ca^{2+} concentration without a concomitant increase in serum phosphorus concentration

Calcitriol acts in concert with PTH to protect against hypocalcemia and hypophosphatemia

The main determinant of serum phosphorus concentration is the ability of the renal proximal tubule to excrete the dietary phosphorus load and conserve phosphorus in the presence of hypophosphatemia

PTH

Bone

In bone, the end result of PTH action is release of phosphorus into the ECF

Small intestine

PTH has no direct effects in intestine

PTH acts indirectly via stimulation of 1-α-hydroxylase to produce calcitriol

Kidney

PTH reduces phosphate reabsorption via its actions in proximal tubule; PTH stimulates endocytic retrieval of Na^+-phosphate cotransporters from the apical membrane

Calcitriol

Bone

Ensures that Ca^{2+} and phosphorus are present in sufficient concentration for bone formation

Potentiates PTH actions

TABLE 10–6 (Continued)
Small intestine
Calcitriol stimulates phosphorus absorption in small intestine where the majority of phosphorus is reabsorbed
Kidney
PTH and hypophosphatemia are the main stimulators of 1-α-hydroxylase and calcitriol production in proximal tubule
Abbreviations: ECF, extracellular fluid; PTH, parathyroid hormone

TABLE 10–7: Renal Phosphorus Excretion—Other Factors

Increase reabsorption

Insulin—inhibits the phosphaturic effect of PTH

Growth hormone—mediated in part by insulin-like growth factor 1 stimulates Na^+-phosphate cotransport

Thyroid hormone—stimulates Na^+-phosphate cotransport

Staniocalcin 1—mediated via the Na^+-phosphate cotransporter

Increase excretion

Calcitonin—reduces Na^+-phosphate cotransport independent of PTH and cyclic AMP

Glucocorticoids—inhibit Na^+-phosphate cotransport independent of PTH

Metabolic acidosis—may be mediated via glucocorticoids

Atrial natriuretic peptide—reduces Na^+-phosphate cotransport

Parathyroid hormone related protein—mechanism identical to PTH

Glucagon

Staniocalcin 2—mediated via the Na^+-phosphate cotransporter

Dopamine—mediated via the Na^+-phosphate cotransporter

Volume expansion—may be related to increases in dopamine and atrial natriuretic peptide

Abbreviations: PTH, parathyroid hormone; AMP, adenosine monophosphate

TABLE 10–8: Phosphorus Regulation—Phosphatonins (Fibroblast Growth Factor-23)
A newly discovered group of compounds that inhibit proximal tubular renal phosphate reabsorption causing hypophosphatemia have been named "phosphatonins"; they do not play a role in regulating serum calcium concentration
Phosphatonins are overproduced by tumors that cause oncogenic osteomalacia
The first two compounds described FGF-23 and sFRP-4 prevent or attenuate the increase in 1-α-hydroxylase activity that would normally occur as a result of hypophosphatemia
FGF-23
FGF-23 plays a role in the pathogenesis of several rare inherited and acquired disorders that present with hypophosphatemia secondary to renal phosphate wasting
Fibroblast growth factor-23 can be detected in the circulation of healthy individuals suggesting it plays a role in normal phosphorus homeostasis
The biologic activity of FGF-23 is limited to the full-length molecule and it is degraded by protease cleavage
Experimental studies in normal animals-phenotype
When administered to animals FGF-23 causes hypophosphatemia, increased renal phosphate excretion, suppression of $1,25(OH)_2$ vitamin D_3, and osteomalacia

(continued)

TABLE 10–8 (Continued)

Studies suggesting that FGF-23 may play a central role in the feedback regulation of calcitriol concentration

FGF-23 when injected into experimental animals reduces calcitriol concentration within 3 h as a result of decreased calcitriol synthesis. Serum phosphorus concentration and NaPi-IIa fall after 9-13 h

This effect is PTH-independent; it is likely that only a part of the phosphaturic effect of FGF-23 is related to decreased calcitriol concentration

Injection of calcitriol into mice results in an increase in FGF-23 concentration and FGF-23 knockout mice have high serum calcitriol concentrations

In humans changes in dietary phosphorus intakes within the physiologic range regulate serum FGF-23 concentration

In normal human volunteers FGF-23 concentration is inversely correlated with serum calcitriol levels

Abbreviations: NaPi, sodium phosphate; FGF, fibroblast growth factor; sFRP, soluble frizzled-related protein

TABLE 10–9: Phosphorus Regulation-Phosphatonins (sFRP-4, MEPE, FGF-7)

sFRP-4

Overexpressed in tumors that cause oncogenic osteomalacia

The purified protein inhibits phosphate transport in a proximal tubular cell line and results in hypophosphatemia when injected into animals

MEPE

Abundantly overexpressed in tumors that cause oncogenic osteomalacia

Increased serum concentration in patients with X-linked hypophosphatemic rickets

Inhibits proximal tubular phosphate reabsorption

Inhibits bone mineralization in vitro

FGF-7

Overexpressed in tumors resulting in oncogenic osteomalacia

Inhibits proximal tubular phosphate transport in cultured proximal tubular cells

Abbreviations: sFRP, soluble frizzled-related protein; MEPE, matrix extracellular phosphoglycoprotein; FGF, fibroblast growth factor

HYPERPHOSPHATEMIA

TABLE 10–10: Etiologies of Hyperphosphatemia
Hyperphosphatemia most commonly results from decreased renal phosphate excretion
Chronic kidney disease is the cause in greater than 90% of cases
Decreased renal excretion
• Decreased glomerular filtration rate
▪ Acute kidney injury
▪ Chronic kidney disease
• Increased renal phosphate reabsorption
▪ Hypoparathyroidism
▪ Acromegaly
▪ Thyrotoxicosis
▪ Drugs—bisphosphonates
▪ Tumoral calcinosis
Acute phosphorus addition to ECF
• Endogenous
▪ Tumor lysis syndrome
▪ Rhabdomyolysis
▪ Severe hemolysis

TABLE 10–10 (Continued)
• Exogenous
■ Vitamin D intoxication
■ Na^+ phosphate-containing bowel preparation solutions
■ High dose liposomal amphotericin B
■ Improperly purified fresh frozen plasma
Pseudohyperphosphatemia
Abbreviation: ECF, extracellular fluid

TABLE 10–11: Hyperphosphatemia—Decreased Renal Phosphorus Excretion

Chronic kidney disease is the most common cause of hyperphosphatemia

Decreased Glomerular Filtration Rate

- Chronic kidney disease

Pathophysiology

As GFR declines below 60 mL/min/1.73 m^2 renal phosphorus excretion increases

Once GFR falls below 30 mL/min/1.73 m^2, phosphate reabsorption is maximally inhibited and renal excretion cannot increase further; dietary intake then exceeds excretion and serum phosphorus concentration increases

A new steady state is established at a higher serum phosphorus concentration

Presentation

Approximately 15% of patients with a GFR of 15–30 mL/min/1.73 m^2 and 50% of those with a GFR < 15 mL/min/1.73 m^2 have hyperphosphatemia

Diagnosis

Measurement of serum blood urea nitrogen and creatinine concentrations

Special patient populations may require 24-h urine creatinine clearance measurements

TABLE 10–11 (Continued)
Increased Renal Phosphate Reabsorption—Uncommon
• Hypoparathyroidism
▪ Decreased PTH concentration or effect
• Acromegaly
▪ Insulin-like growth factor stimulates phosphate transport in proximal tubule
• Drugs—bisphosphonates
▪ Directly increases renal phosphate reabsorption but this effect is usually offset by secondary hyperparathyroidism resulting from hypocalcemia
• Tumoral calcinosis
▪ Autosomal recessive disease associated with hyperphosphatemia and soft tissue Ca^{2+} deposition caused by mutations in two genes
▪ Inactivating mutations of GALNT3 which encodes a glycosyltransferase involved in O-linked glycosylation
▪ An FGF-23 mutation was identified that affects a serine residue that may be involved in FGF-23 glycosylation
▪ It was hypothesized that GALNT3 controls FGF-23 glycosylation and that glycosylation may be required for normal FGF-23 function
Abbreviation: GFR, glomerular filtration rate

TABLE 10–12: Hyperphosphatemia—Phosphorus Addition to ECF (Endogenous Source)

- Tumor lysis syndrome

Pathophysiology

Malignant lymphoid cells contain up to four times as much phosphorus as normal lymphocytes

Precipitation of uric acid results in acute kidney injury-urate nephropathy

Precipitation of calcium phosphate can result in acute nephrocalcinosis and acute kidney injury

Presentation

Seen classically with treatment of Burkitt's lymphoma or acute lymphocytic leukemia

Characterized by hyperphosphatemia, hypocalcemia, hyperuricemia, and hyperkalemia

Acute kidney injury is a common consequence

Hyperphosphatemia classically occurs about 24–48 h after onset of chemotherapy

Can occur in patients with solid tumors when there is a decrease in GFR or tumor burden is large; an increased LDH concentration (>1500 IU), hyperuricemia, large tumor burden and high tumor sensitivity to treatment are predictive of the development of tumor lysis syndrome with solid tumors

Treatment

Prevention of acute urate nephropathy is directed at reducing uric acid formation or converting it to a more soluble compound to facilitate its renal excretion

TABLE 10–12 (Continued)

Higher primates do not express urate oxidase that converts uric acid to the more soluble allantoin
Purines are metabolized to hypoxanthine and xanthine; xanthine is then converted to uric acid by xanthine oxidase, which is inhibited by allopurinol (half-life of 0.5–2.0 h)
Allopurinol is metabolized to oxypurinol that also inhibits xanthine oxidase but is renally excreted with a half-life of 18–30 h
Allopurinol must be used with caution in patients with decreased GFR
Uric acid can be converted to the more soluble sodium urate by increasing urinary pH to 6.5 with sodium bicarbonate; this must be done with caution because calcium phosphate precipitation increases at urinary pHs > 6.5
Recombinant urate oxidase (rasburicase) was recently approved by the FDA; it cannot be used in patients with glucose-6-phosphate dehydrogenase deficiency since hydrogen peroxide generated during allantoin formation may cause hemolysis
• Hemolysis
• Rhabdomyolysis

Abbreviations: ECF, extracellular fluid; GFR, glomerular filtration rate; LDH, lactate dehydrogenase; FDA, Food and Drug Administration

TABLE 10–13: Hyperphosphatemia—Phosphorus Addition to ECF (Exogenous Source)
• Oral sodium phosphate-containing laxatives and enemas
Oral sodium phosphate solution is commonly used as a bowel preparation agent for colonoscopy
It can be given in a small volume (45 mL 18 and 6 h before the procedure) and is less expensive than polyethylene glycol-based solutions
Ninety mL contain 43.2 g of monobasic sodium phosphate and 16.2 g of dibasic sodium phosphate
Its use can result in severe hyperphosphatemia, acute kidney injury, and death
Pathophysiology
Acute kidney injury occurs as a result of nephrocalcinosis
Presentation
Fatal hyperphosphatemia was reported in a renal transplant patient, serum phosphorus concentration 17.8 mg/dL, who received a single oral dose of 90 mL and suffered a cardiorespiratory arrest 6 h later; four other deaths were reported; two of these four patients had end-stage renal disease
The rise in serum phosphorus concentration that occurs after ingestion of oral sodium phosphate is directly correlated with patient age
The majority of reported patients were women and in one series 90% of those affected were taking either angiotensin-converting enzyme inhibitors or angiotensin-receptor blockers

TABLE 10–13 (Continued)
Treatment
Oral sodium phosphate solution should be used with caution in those above age 55, those with decreased gastrointestinal motility, patients with decreased GFR, and in the presence of volume depletion
Renal dysfunction is often irreversible
• Vitamin D intoxication
• High dose liposomal amphotericin (phosphatidylcholine, phosphatidylserine)
• Solvent detergent treated fresh frozen plasma
■ Contained improper amounts of dihydrogen phosphate used as a buffer in the purification process
Abbreviations: ECF, extracellular fluid; GFR, glomerular filtration rate

TABLE 10–14: Signs and Symptoms

Signs and symptoms of hyperphosphatemia are primarily the result of hypocalcemia (see previous chapter)

Pathophysiology of hypocalcemia induced by hyperphosphatemia

The most common explanation offered for hypocalcemia is that the calcium phosphorus product exceeds a certain level and Ca^{2+} deposits in soft tissues and serum Ca^{2+} concentration falls

Calcium phosphorus product of > 72 mg/dL is commonly believed to result in "metastatic" calcification

Short-term infusions of phosphorus increase bone Ca^{2+} deposition and reduce bone resorption

Hypocalcemia can also result from decreased calcitriol concentration from suppression of 1-α-hydroxylase by increased serum phosphorus; these effects may be more important than physicochemical precipitation

The hypothesis that hypocalcemia results from soft tissue deposition is inconsistent with the observation in experimental animals that serum Ca^{2+} concentration continues to decline for up to 5 days after phosphorus infusions are discontinued and long beyond the time period when serum phosphorus concentration normalizes

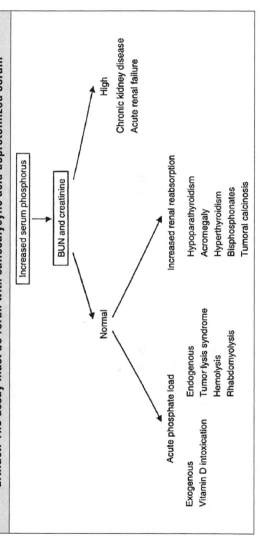

FIGURE 10–2: An Algorithm for the Approach to the Patient with Hyperphosphatemia. The cause is generally acute kidney injury or chronic kidney disease. Unexplained persistent hyperphosphatemia should raise the suspicion of pseudohyperphosphatemia, the most common cause is paraproteinemia secondary to multiple myeloma. No consistent relationship of immunoglobulin type or subclass was identified. This is a method-dependent artifact. The assay must be rerun with sulfosalycylic acid deproteinized serum

TABLE 10–15: Treatment

The cornerstone of treatment is reduction of intestinal phosphorus absorption

Dietary phosphorus restriction

Early in chronic kidney disease hyperphosphatemia can be controlled with dietary phosphorus restriction

Dietary phosphorus absorption is linear over a wide range of intakes (4–30 mg/kg/day) and absorption depends on the amount of dietary phosphorus and its bioavailability

The majority of dietary phosphorus is contained in three food groups: (1) milk and related dairy products such as cheese; (2) meat, poultry, and fish; and (3) grains

Processed foods may contain large amounts of phosphorus; in one study an additional 1154 mg/day of phosphorus was ingested secondary to phosphorus-containing additives in fast food with no change in dietary protein intake

Phosphorus contained in plants is largely in the form of phytate and has low bioavailability since humans do not express intestinal phytase that is necessary to degrade phytate and release phosphorus

Phosphorus in meats and dairy products is well absorbed

Inorganic phosphorus salts in processed foods are virtually completely absorbed and patients with hyperphosphatemia should avoid these foods including hot dogs, cheese spreads, colas, processed meats, and instant puddings

Dietary estimates of phosphorus ingestion commonly underestimate phosphorus intake

TABLE 10–15 (Continued)

Phosphate binders

As chronic kidney disease worsens phosphate binders must be added

The optimal choice of a phosphate binder remains controversial

The ideal binder should efficiently bind phosphate, have minimal effects on comorbid conditions, have a favorable side-effect profile, and be low in cost; none of the currently available binders fulfill all of these criteria

Ca^{2+}-containing binders are low in cost but may contribute to net positive Ca^{2+} balance and vascular Ca^{2+} deposition

Aluminum-containing binders can be employed in the short term but should be avoided chronically because of aluminum toxicity (osteomalacia and dementia)

Sevelamer HCl, a synthetic Ca^{2+}-free polymer, has a favorable side-effect profile but is costly

Lanthanum carbonate was recently approved by the FDA; it is costly and associated with significant GI toxicity

The hyperphosphatemic patient with coexistent hypocalcemia

It is preferable to first lower serum phosphorus concentration below 6 mg/dL, if possible, before treating the hypocalcemia

This is not always possible and clinical judgment must be used

Abbreviations: GI, gastrointestinal; FDA, Food and Drug Administration

HYPOPHOSPHATEMIA

TABLE 10–16: Etiologies of Hypophosphatemia
Decreased intestinal absorption
Decreased dietary intake
Phosphate-binding agents
Alcoholism
Redistribution from extracellular to intracellular fluid
Respiratory alkalosis
Refeeding
Diabetic ketoacidosis
Hungry bone syndrome
Sepsis
Increased renal excretion
Primary hyperparathyroidism
Secondary hyperparathyroidism from vitamin D deficiency with intact renal function
X-linked hypophophatemic rickets
Autosomal dominant hypophosphatemic rickets
Oncogenic osteomalacia
Fibrous dysplasia of bone

TABLE 10–16 (Continued)
Hereditary hypophosphatemic rickets with hypercalciuria
Imatinib mesylate
Fanconi's syndrome
Osmotic diuresis
Hepatic resection
Pseudohypophosphatemia

TABLE 10–17: Hypophosphatemia-Extrarenal Causes (Cell Shift)

Shift of phosphorus from ECF to intracellular fluid

Respiratory Alkalosis

Pathophysiology

The rise in intracellular pH that occurs with respiratory alkalosis stimulates phosphofructokinase, the rate-limiting step in glycolysis, and phosphorus moves intracellularly and is incorporated into ATP

Presentation

Severe hypophosphatemia with phosphorus concentrations less than 0.5–1.0 mg/dL is common

The most common cause of hypophosphatemia in hospitalized patients

Hypophosphatemia was reported with a rise in pH even within the normal range in ventilated chronic obstructive pulmonary disease patients; in concert with the rise in pH that occurs after intubation serum phosphorus concentration falls over the span of several hours

Refeeding Syndrome

Pathophysiology

Carbohydrate repletion and insulin release enhance intracellular uptake of phosphorus, glucose, and K^+

The combination of total body phosphorus depletion from decreased intake and increased cellular uptake during refeeding leads to profound hypophosphatemia

TABLE 10–17 (Continued)
Presentation
With refeeding the time of onset of hypophosphatemia depends on the degree of malnutrition, caloric load, and amount of phosphorus in the formulation; in undernourished patients it develops in 2–5 days
Hypophosphatemia can occur with both enteral and parenteral refeeding
The fall in serum phosphorus concentration is more marked with liver disease
In adolescents with anorexia nervosa the fall in serum phosphorus concentration is directly proportional to the percent loss of ideal body weight
Serum phosphorus concentration rarely declines below 0.5 mg/dL with glucose infusion alone
Treatment of Diabetic Ketoacidosis
Insulin administration results in phosphorus movement into cells
Renal phosphate loss from osmotic diuresis also contributes
Post Partial Parathyroidectomy for Secondary Hyperparathyroidism—"Hungry Bone Syndrome"
Serum Ca^{2+} and phosphorus concentration often fall abruptly in the immediate postoperative period
From a clinical standpoint hypocalcemia is the more important management issue
Patients should be observed carefully for hyperkalemia with Ca^{2+} replacement in the postoperative period

(continued)

TABLE 10–17 (Continued)
Sepsis
Catecholamines and cytokines may also cause a phosphorus shift into cells and this may be the mechanism whereby sepsis results in hypophosphatemia
Abbreviations: ECF, extracellular fluid; ATP, adenosine triphosphate

TABLE 10–18: Hypophosphatemia—Extrarenal Causes (GI)
Decreased intestinal absorption
Decreased GI absorption alone is an uncommon cause of hypophosphatemia since dietary phosphorus intake invariably exceeds GI losses and the kidney is extraordinarily effective at conserving phosphorus decreased dietary intake must be combined with the use of phosphate binders or increased GI losses as with diarrhea
• Decreased dietary intake
• Phosphate-binding agents
• Alcoholism
Abbreviation: GI, gastrointestinal

TABLE 10–19: Hypophosphatemia—Increased Renal Phosphate Excretion (Selective Lesion—PTH Related)

Secondary to an increased concentration of parathyroid hormone

Primary Hyperparathyroidism

Pathophysiology

Parathyroid hormone stimulates endocytic retrieval of Na^+-phosphate cotransporters from the luminal membrane of the proximal tubular cell

Presentation

Although PTH increases renal phosphate excretion, this is partially offset by PTH action to increase calcitriol that in turn increases GI phosphorus absorption, and PTH effect in bone that results in phosphorus release

Serum phosphorus concentration is rarely below 1.5 mg/dL

Secondary Hyperparathyroidism from Disorders of Vitamin D Metabolism

Pathophysiology

Secondary hyperparathyroidism from calcitriol deficiency may be associated with severe hypophosphatemia if the patient has normal renal function

Presentation

Can present with severe hypophosphatemia

Abbreviations: PTH, parathyroid hormone; GI, gastrointestinal

TABLE 10–20: Hypophosphatemia—Increased Renal Phosphate Excretion (Selective Lesion-Phosphatonin Related)

XLH
Pathophysiology
X-linked dominant disorder with a prevalence of 1:20,000
XLH is caused by mutations in the PHEX gene
PHEX is expressed in bone, teeth, and parathyroid gland but not in kidney
In bone, PHEX is expressed in the osteoblast cell membrane and plays a role in mineralization
The mutated protein is not expressed in the cell membrane and is degraded in endoplasmic reticulum
PHEX may play a role in the activation or inactivation of peptide factors involved in skeletal mineralization, renal phosphate transport, and vitamin D metabolism
Elevated concentrations of FGF-23 and MEPE were described
Presentation
Growth retardation, rickets, hypophosphatemia, renal phosphate wasting, and low serum calcitriol concentration

TABLE 10–20 (Continued)

ADHR

Pathophysiology

Mutations in FGF-23 cause ADHR

FGF-23, a 251-amino acid protein, is secreted and processed at a cleavage site into inactive N- and C-terminal fragments; mutations in ADHR occur at the proteolytic site and prevent cleavage

Presentation

ADHR has a similar phenotype to XLH but is inherited in an autosomal dominant fashion with variable penetrance

OOM

Pathophysiology

OOM is caused by overproduction of FGF-23, MEPE and possibly other phosphatonins produced by mesenchymal tumors

Presentation

Hypophosphatemia, renal phosphate wasting, suppression of 1-α-hydroxylase and osteomalacia

The tumor is often difficult to localize

Tumor resection is curative; immunohistochemical staining shows an overabundance of FGF-23

Fibrous Dysplasia of Bone—Rare

Pathophysiology

In the subset of patients with hypophosphatemia FGF-23 levels are elevated

(continued)

TABLE 10–20 (Continued)
The result of somatic activating missense mutations of GNAS1 which encodes the alpha subunit of the stimulatory G protein, G_s

Presentation
McCune-Albright Syndrome—triad of precocious puberty, café au lait spots, and fibrous dysplasia of bone
Can involve oversecretion of other hormones—thyroid hormone, parathyroid hormone, pituitary hormones
Congenital disorder presenting with bone pain, deformity, and fracture involving one (monostotic) or multiple (polyostotic) bones

Abbreviations: XLH, X-linked hypophosphatemic rickets; PHEX, phosphate regulating gene with homology to endopeptidases; FGF, fibroblast growth factor; ADHR, autosomal dominant hypophosphatemic rickets; OOM, oncogenic osteomalacia; MEPE, matrix extracellular phosphoglycoprotein

TABLE 10–21: Hypophosphatemia—Increased Renal Phosphate Excretion (Selective Lesion—Miscellaneous)

HHRH
Autosomal recessive inheritance
Secondary to a loss of function mutation in the sodium-phosphate cotransporter gene SLC34A3
Presents with hypophosphatemia, rickets, and reduced renal phosphate reabsorption
Calcitriol levels are increased
Imatinib mesylate
Tyrosine kinase inhibitor
Hypophosphatemia due to increased renal phosphate excretion in patients treated for CML and gastrointestinal stromal tumors
Imatinib through its inhibiton of tyrosine kinases may interfere with osteoclast and osteoblast function
Abbreviation: HHRH, hereditary hypophosphatemic rickets with hypercalciuria; CML, chronic myelogenous leukemia

TABLE 10–22: Hypophosphatemia—Increased Renal Phosphate Excretion (Nonselective Lesion)

Fanconi's Syndrome

Pathophysiology

Caused by a variety of disorders that result in a generalized proximal tubular transport defect

Inherited—Cystinosis, Wilson's disease, hereditary fructose intolerance, and Lowe's syndrome

Acquired—Multiple myeloma, renal transplantation, and drugs

Drugs—Ifosfamide, streptozocin, tetracyclines, valproic acid, ddI, cidofovir, adefovir, tenofovir, and ranitidine

Presentation

Renal phosphate wasting, glycosuria in the face of a normal serum glucose concentration, and aminoaciduria

Less commonly patients may also have proximal renal tubular acidosis and hypokalemia

Diagnosis

A urinalysis for glycosuria should be performed

The diagnosis is established by measuring serum and urinary amino acids and glucose and calculating the fractional excretion of each

Fanconi's Syndrome Secondary to Tenofovir

Pathophysiology

Tenofovir is an acyclic nucleoside phosphonate that is excreted by glomerular filtration and tubular secretion

TABLE 10–22 (Continued)
It enters the tubular cell across the basolateral membrane on the hOAT1 and exits into the urine on the Mrp2
Since ritonavir inhibits Mrp2, its use with tenofovir could result in increased toxicity
Presentation
Injury occurs weeks to months after starting treatment
Decreases in creatinine clearance and nephrogenic diabetes insipidus were also reported
Dent's Disease
Pathophysiology
Caused by a mutation in the Cl⁻ channel CLCN 5
Presentation
Hypophosphatemia and renal phosphate wasting associated with low molecular weight proteinuria, hypercalciuria, nephrolithiasis, nephrocalcinosis, and chronic kidney disease
Chinese Herb Boui-ougi-tou
Used for the treatment of obesity
Renal damage may be related to aristocholic acid
Abbreviations: hOAT1, human organic anion transporter 1; Mrp2, multi resistant-associated protein 2; CLCN5, chloride channel 5; PTH, parathyroid hormone; GI, gastrointestinal; MEPE, matrix extracellular phosphoglycoprotein

TABLE 10–23: Signs and Symptoms
Hypophosphatemia causes a variety of signs and symptoms; their severity varies with the degree of phosphorus lowering
Moderate hypophosphatemia—(serum phosphorus concentration 1.0–2.5 mg/dL)
With the exception of the respiratory system there is little evidence that moderate hypophosphatemia (phosphorus concentration 1.0–2.5 mg/dL) results in any clinically significant morbidity
Correction improved diaphragmatic function in patients with acute respiratory failure
In two studies patients with moderate hypophosphatemia had an increase in ventricular arrhythmias; there was no increase in mortality; more studies are needed to address this issue
Moderate hypophosphatemia does not impair cardiac contractility
Moderate hypophosphatemia increases insulin resistance but the clinical significance of this is unclear
Severe hypophosphatemia (serum phosphorus concentration <1.0 mg/dL) is associated with morbidity
Failure to wean from mechanical ventilation without correction of severe hypophosphatemia was demonstrated
Severe hypophosphatemia produces reversible myocardial dysfunction and an impaired response to pressors

TABLE 10–23 (Continued)

Hematologic disturbances include increases in red cell fragility that lead to clinically significant hemolysis; associated with reduced red cell ATP levels and large declines in hemoglobin concentration and hematocrit; serum phosphorus concentration is often very low (≤ 0.2 mg/dL)

Hypophosphatemia causes a leftward shift in the oxygen dissociation curve of unclear clinical significance

A variety of neuromuscular symptoms were reported including paresthesias, tremor, and muscle weakness

Severe hypophosphatemia causes rhabdomyolysis in dogs only if there is a preexisting subclinical myopathy; there are case reports associated with severe hypophosphatemia in alcoholics

Abbreviation: ATP, adenosine triphosphate

$$\frac{U_P \times P_{Cr}}{U_{Cr} \times P_P} \times 100 \qquad (10\text{-}1)$$

Formula for the fractional excretion (FE) of phosphorus

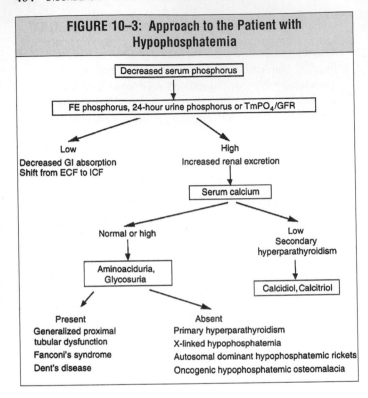

FIGURE 10–3: Approach to the Patient with Hypophosphatemia

TABLE 10–24: Approach to the Patient with a Low Serum Phosphorus Concentration

The most common cause of hypophosphatemia in hospitalized patients is the result of phosphorus shift into cells secondary to respiratory alkalosis

Primary and secondary hyperparathyroidism are the most common causes of renal phosphate wasting

Step 1 Evaluate renal phosphorus handling

One can use the FE of phosphorus, 24-h urinary phosphorus, or calculated renal threshold phosphate concentration ($TmPO_4$/GFR) to determine the kidneys response to hypophosphatemia

A FE of phosphorus below 5% or a 24-h urine phosphorus less than 100 mg/day indicates that the kidney is responding properly to decreased intestinal absorption or shift of phosphorus into cells

If renal phosphorus wasting is the pathophysiologic reason for hypophosphatemia, then the FE of phosphorus exceeds 5% and 24-h urine phosphate excretion is greater than 100 mg

Step 2 In the patient with increased renal phosphate excretion one next evaluates the serum Ca^{2+} concentration

- Serum Ca^{2+} concentration low

- Secondary hyperparathyroidism from disorders of vitamin D metabolism (normal renal function)

    ▪ Calcidiol and calcitriol concentrations help identify the defect

TABLE 10–24 (Continued)
• Serum Ca^{2+} concentration normal or high
■ Isolated renal phosphate wasting—no glycosuria or aminoaciduria
■ Primary hyperparathyroidism is by far the most common diagnosis
■ Associated with high serum Ca^{2+} concentration and low serum phosphorus concentration
■ Diagnosis established by measuring PTH concentration
■ Rare inherited and acquired disorders related to phosphatonins
■ X-linked hypophosphatemic rickets
■ Autosomal dominant hypophosphatemic rickets
■ Oncogenic osteomalacia
■ Fibrous dysplasia of bone
■ Generalized proximal tubular disorder—associated with aminoaciduria and glycosuria
■ Fanconi's syndrome
■ Dent's disease
Pseudohypophosphatemia
Suspect if severe hypophosphatemia is noted without symptoms or serum phosphorus concentration remains low despite repletion
As in the case with pseudohyperphosphatemia paraproteins can also result in a spuriously low serum phosphorus concentration
Can be avoided if deproteinized serum is analyzed
Abbreviations: FE, fractional excretion; PTH, parathyroid hormone

TABLE 10–25: Treatment

There is little evidence that treatment of moderate hypophosphatemia (serum phosphorus concentration 1.0–2.5 mg/dL) is necessary except perhaps in the mechanically ventilated patient

Severe hypophosphatemia (≤ 1 mg/dL) or its symptoms are indications for treatment

In the severely malnourished patient, such as an adolescent with anorexia nervosa, refeeding must be accomplished slowly; serum phosphorus concentration should be monitored closely and the patient placed on telemetry since sudden death and ventricular arrhythmias were reported with refeeding

General principles

Hypophosphatemia is commonly associated with other electrolyte disturbances (hypokalemia and hypomagnesemia)

One must cautiously replete phosphorus in patients that have impaired ability to excrete phosphorus loads (those with decreased GFR) and in patients that are hypocalcemic

One must keep in mind that serum phosphorus concentration may not be a reliable indicator of total body phosphorus stores since the majority of phosphorus is contained within cells

Oral repletion

Most hypophosphatemic patients can be corrected with up to 1 g of supplemental phosphorus per day orally; several forms of oral phosphorus replacement are listed in Table 10–26

Oral repletion is most commonly limited by diarrhea

(continued)

TABLE 10–25 (Continued)
IV phosphorus administration
IV phosphate administration may be complicated by hypocalcemia and hyperphosphatemia and is only justified in those with severe symptomatic phosphorus depletion
Sodium phosphate should be employed except in patients that require concomitant K^+ supplementation
During IV replacement blood chemistries including serum phosphorus, Ca^{2+}, Mg^{2+}, and K^+ should be monitored closely
Once serum phosphorus concentration has risen above 1 mg/dL, an oral preparation is begun and IV phosphorus discontinued
Abbreviations: IV, intravenous; GFR, glomerular filtration rate

TABLE 10–26: Phosphorus Replacement (Oral)			
Preparation	**Phosphorus**	**Sodium**	**Potassium**
KPhos neutral	250 mg/tab	13 mEq/tab	1.1 mEq/tab
KPhos original	114 mg/tab	None	3.7 mEq/tab
Fleets phospho-soda	129 mg/mL	4.8 mEq/mL	None
Neutra-phos-K	250 mg/cap	None	13.6 mEq/cap
Neutra-phos	250 mg/cap	7.1 mEq/cap	6.8 mEq/cap
Abbreviation: IV, intravenous			

	TABLE 10–27: Phosphorus Replacement (IV)			
Preparation	**Phosphorus (mg/mL)**	**Phosphorus (mmol/mL)**	**Sodium**	**Potassium**
IV Na^+ phosphate	93	3	4.0 mEq/mL	None
IV K^+ phosphate	93	3	None	4.4 mEq/mL
Abbreviation: IV, intravenous				

TABLE 10–28: Phosphorus Replacement Protocols (IV)

A variety of rapid repletion protocols were used safely. Do not use these protocols in patients with hypocalcemia or stage 4 or 5 CKD

Author	Dose	Degree of Hypophosphatemia
Rosen	15 mmol over 2h Q6h, no > 45 mmol/day total	moderate
Vannatta	9 mmol Q12h for 48 h	severe
Vannatta	0.32–0.48 mmol/kg Q12 h for 48 h	severe
Kingston	0.25 mmol/kg over 4 h ([P]: 0.5 mg/dL–1.0 mg/dL) 0.50 mmol/kg over 4 h ([P]: < 0.5 mg/dL)	severe
Perreault	15 mmol over 3 h ([P]:1.27 mg/dL–2.48 mg/dL) 30 mmol over 3 h ([P]: < 1.24 mg/dL)	moderate severe
Charron	30 mmol over 2–4 h ([P]:1.25 mg/dL –2.03 mg/dL) 45 mmol over 3–6 h ([P]: < 1.25 mg/dL)	moderate severe
Taylor	10 mmol: 40–60 kg, 15 mmol: 61–80 kg, 20 mmol: 81–120 kg ([P]:1.8 mg/dL –22 mg/dL) 20 mmol:40–60 kg, 30 mmol: 61–80 kg, 40 mmol: 81–120 kg ([P]: 1.0–1.7 mg/dL) 30 mmol: 40–60 kg, 40 mmol: 61–120 kg, 50 mmol: 81–120 kg ([P]: <1.0 mg/dL) Infusions given over 6 h	mild moderate severe

Abbreviations: IV, intravenous; [P], serum phosphorus concentration

11
Disorders of Serum Magnesium

INTRODUCTION

TABLE 11–1: Magnesium Homeostasis—Overview
Magnesium is the fourth most abundant cation in the body and second most abundant within cells
Normal serum magnesium concentration is between 1.7 and 2.5 mg/dL (1.2–1.75 mEq/L, 0.6–0.9 mmol/L)
Magnesium plays a key role in a variety of cellular processes
• Magnesium is an important cofactor for ATPases and thereby, in the maintenance of intracellular electrolyte composition
• Ion channels involved in nerve conduction and cardiac contractility are regulated by Mg^{2+}
• Over 300 enzymatic systems depend on magnesium for optimal function including those involved in protein synthesis and DNA replication
• Mg^{2+} deficiency is implicated in the pathogenesis of hypertension, type II diabetes mellitus, atherosclerosis, and asthma
Only 1% of the 21–28 g of Mg^{2+} in the body is contained within the ECF; of the remainder, 67% is in bone and 20% in muscle
Abbreviations: ATP, adenosine triphosphate; DNA, deoxyribonucleic acid; ECF, extracellular fluid

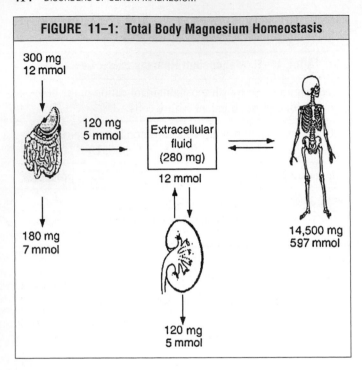

FIGURE 11–1: Total Body Magnesium Homeostasis

300 mg
12 mmol

120 mg
5 mmol

Extracellular fluid
(280 mg)

12 mmol

180 mg
7 mmol

14,500 mg
597 mmol

120 mg
5 mmol

TABLE 11–2: Magnesium Fluxes between ECF and Organ Systems

Mg^{2+} is regulated by both GI tract and kidney, with kidney playing the most important role

The average North American diet contains 200–350 mg of magnesium

- The average daily requirement in men is 220–400 mg and in women is 180–340 mg

- The North American diet is only marginally adequate with respect to magnesium

Magnesium absorption is inversely proportional to intake

- Normally 30–40% is absorbed; this can vary from 25% to 80%

- The majority of Mg^{2+} absorption occurs in small intestine via both a paracellular and transcellular pathway

- Magnesium absorption is affected by water absorption and prolonged diarrheal states result in significant magnesium losses

- Secretions from the upper GI tract are relatively low in magnesium (1 mg/dL) while those from colon are relatively high in magnesium (18 mg/dL)

The primary regulator of ECF magnesium concentration is the kidney

- Renal magnesium reabsorption varies widely to maintain homeostasis

- Reabsorption is reduced to near zero in the presence of hypermagnesemia or CKD

- With magnesium depletion secondary to GI causes the FE of magnesium can be reduced to 0.5%

Abbreviations: ECF, extracellular fluid; GI, gastrointestinal; CKD, chronic kidney disease; FE, fractional excretion

TABLE 11–3: Renal Magnesium Handling—Proximal Tubule and Thick Ascending Limb

Only 30% of Mg^{2+} is bound to albumin; the remainder is freely filtered across the glomerulus

Proximal tubule

Fifteen percent is reabsorbed in the proximal tubule in adults

- ECF volume status affects magnesium reabsorption in this segment

- Volume contraction increases and volume expansion decreases magnesium reabsorption

Thick ascending limb (Figure 11–2)

The bulk of Mg^{2+} reabsorption occurs in cortical thick ascending limb (70%)

- Mg^{2+} is reabsorbed paracellularly with the lumen-positive voltage acting as driving force

- The voltage is generated by K^+ exit across the apical membrane through the ROMK channel

- Mg^{2+} moves across the tight junction through a specific channel, paracellin-1, that transports Mg^{2+} and Ca^{2+}

- The Mg^{2+} concentration sensed at the basolateral surface of the cortical thick ascending limb is the major determinant of Mg^{2+} reabsorption

- In hypermagnesemic states Mg^{2+} reabsorption approaches zero and in hypomagnesemia the loop reabsorbs virtually all of the filtered Mg^{2+} reaching it

TABLE 11-3 (Continued)

- This effect is mediated via the Ca^{2+}-Mg^{2+}-sensing receptor expressed along the thick ascending limb basolateral surface; the receptor senses elevated Ca^{2+} and Mg^{2+} concentration and transduces this signal to the apical membrane resulting in an inhibition of the Na^+-K^+-$2Cl^-$ cotransporter and K^+ recycling; this dissipates the lumen-positive voltage and decreases the driving force for Mg^{2+} reabsorption

Abbreviations: ECF, extracellular fluid; ROMK, renal outer medullary potassium

FIGURE 11-2: Magnesium Reabsorption in the Thick Ascending Limb

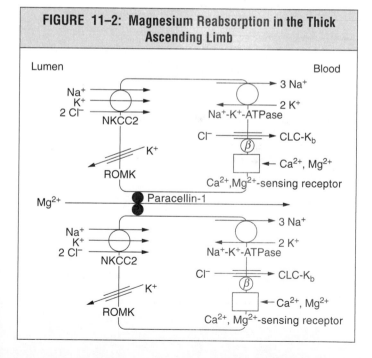

TABLE 11–4: Renal Magnesium Handling—Distal Convoluted Tubule (Figure 11–3)

Approximately 10% of magnesium is reabsorbed in distal convoluted tubule; magnesium transport here is active and transcellular

- Magnesium enters the cell passively through a channel (TRPM6) and exits actively via an unknown mechanism

- Despite differences in transport mechanisms compared to thick ascending limb, hypomagnesemia increases Mg^{2+} reabsorption in this segment

- Amiloride increases Mg^{2+} reabsorption in the distal nephron and is used therapeutically to reduce renal Mg^{2+} loss

- Thiazide diuretics, on the other hand, cause mild Mg^{2+} wasting; distal Mg^{2+} loss is partially offset by increased proximal reabsorption due to mild ECF volume contraction

The collecting duct plays a very limited role

Abbreviations: ECF, extracellular fluid; TRP, transient receptor potential

FIGURE 11–3: Magnesium Reabsorption in the Distal Convoluted Tubule. Mg^{2+} crosses the apical membrane of epithelial cells in intestine and distal nephron via a channel (TRPM6). The exit pathway is unknown

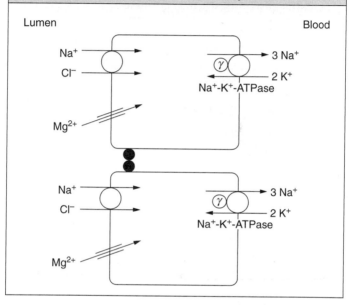

HYPOMAGNESEMIA

TABLE 11–5: Etiologies of Hypomagnesemia
Increased gastrointestinal Mg^{2+} losses
Decreased oral intake
Malabsorption
Diarrhea
Primary intestinal hypomagnesemia
Increased renal Mg^{2+} losses
Primary
• Drugs
• Toxins
• Miscellaneous tubular injury
• Genetic disorders
Secondary
• Osmotic diuresis
• Saline infusion
• Diuretics
• Hypercalcemia
• Metabolic acidosis
Magnesium shifts from extracellular to intracellular space
Hungry bone syndrome
Refeeding syndrome
Hyperthyroidism

TABLE 11-6: Hypomagnesemia—Extrarenal Causes (GI)

Decreased oral intake

- Clinically significant Mg^{2+} depletion from decreased oral intake alone is rare due to the ubiquitous nature of Mg^{2+} in foods and the kidney's ability to conserve Mg^{2+}

Increased GI losses

- Malabsorption

  - Serum Mg^{2+} concentration in these patients tends to correlate with the degree of steatorrhea

  - Presumably intestinal free fatty acids bind Mg^{2+} forming insoluble soaps

  - Mg^{2+} malabsorption improves with a low-fat diet

- Diarrhea

  - Fecal Mg^{2+} increases as stool water increases and colonic secretions are high in Mg^{2+}

- Primary intestinal hypomagnesemia

  - Autosomal recessive disorder characterized by hypomagnesemia and hypocalcemia

  - Patients present in the first 6 months of life with symptoms of neuromuscular excitability including seizures secondary to hypomagnesemia and hypocalcemia

  - The hypocalcemia is resistant to therapy with Ca^{2+} or vitamin D analogues

  - Passive intestinal Mg^{2+} transport is normal and large doses of oral Mg^{2+} reverse the hypomagnesemia and hypocalcemia

(continued)

TABLE 11–6 (Continued)
■ Mutations in the TRPM6 gene cause this disorder; TRPM6 is a member of the TRP channel family and is expressed in intestine and distal nephron; TRPM6 is the pathway whereby Mg^{2+} crosses the apical membrane of epithelial cells in intestine and distal nephron
Abbreviations: GI, gastrointestinal; TRP, transient receptor potential

TABLE 11–7: Hypomagnesemia—Extrarenal Causes (Cell Shift)
Magnesium shift from ECF to intracellular fluid
• Post parathyroidectomy
• Refeeding
• Hyperthyroidism
Mg^{2+} loss from skin
• Burn patient
■ Mg^{2+} loss is proportional to the area burned
Abbreviation: ECF, extracellular fluid

TABLE 11–8: Hypomagnesemia—Renal Causes

Primary renal defects are more likely to cause severe hypomagnesemia than secondary defects

Drug- or toxin-induced injury is the most common cause of renal Mg^{2+} wasting

Primary defects in renal tubular Mg^{2+} reabsorption

- Drug or toxin-induced injury

  - Offending drugs include aminoglycosides, *cis*-platinum, amphotericin B, pentamidine, cyclosporin, tacrolimus, and cetuximab

  - With *cis*-platinum hypomagnesemia may persist for years after the drug is discontinued

  - Cyclosporin-induced hypomagnesemia is often associated with normal or elevated serum K^+ concentration and resolves rapidly after discontinuation of the drug

  - Hypomagnesemia may occur up to 2 weeks after a course of pentamidine

- Tubular damage

  - Acute tubular necrosis

  - Post urinary tract obstruction

  - Delayed renal allograft function

- Inherited disorders (see Table 11–9)

(continued)

TABLE 11–8 (Continued)
Systemic and local factors that affect renal Mg^{2+} reabsorption
• Osmotic diuresis
▪ Reduced proximal tubular Mg^{2+} reabsorption
• Saline infusion
▪ Reduced proximal tubular Mg^{2+} reabsorption
• Loop diuretics
▪ Inhibit Mg^{2+} reabsorption in the loop of Henle
▪ This effect is mild due to an associated increase in proximal reabsorption
• Hypercalcemia
▪ Ca binds to the Ca^{2+}-Mg^{2+} receptor in the basolateral membrane of the loop of Henle decreasing the lumen-positive voltage that drives paracellular Mg^{2+} transport
• Metabolic acidosis
▪ Downregulates TRPM6
• Thiazide diuretics
▪ Act in distal convoluted tubule to inhibit Mg^{2+} transport
▪ Downregulate TRPM6 expression in the luminal membrane of DCT
Abbreviation: DCT, distal convoluted tubule

TABLE 11–9: Hypomagnesemia— Hereditary Renal Causes (Thick Ascending Limb, Figure 11–2)

These disorders are uncommon

They are differentiated based on whether they are associated with hypercalciuria (thick ascending limb defects) or hypocalciuria (distal convoluted tubule defects)

FHHNC

Pathophysiology

Mutations in paracellin 1 cause FHHNC

Paracellin 1 is expressed in the tight junction of the thick ascending limb of Henle; it may function as a paracellular Ca^{2+}- and Mg^{2+}-selective channel

Presentation

Characterized by renal Mg^{2+} and Ca^{2+} wasting

It presents in early childhood with recurrent urinary tract infections, nephrolithiasis, and a urinary concentrating defect

The associated hypercalciuria, incomplete distal renal tubular acidosis, and hypocitraturia result in nephrocalcinosis and a progressive decrease in glomerular filtration rate

One-third develop end-stage renal disease by early adolescence

ADH

Pathophysiology

In ADH and Bartter syndrome the driving force stimulating passive Mg^{2+} transport (lumen-positive voltage) is dissipated

(continued)

TABLE 11–9 (Continued)
ADH results from an activating mutation in the Ca^{2+}-Mg^{2+}-sensing receptor
Activating mutations increase receptor affinity for Ca^{2+} and Mg^{2+}; this signal is transduced to the apical membrane resulting in an inhibition of apical Na^+ entry and K^+ exit
The reduction in lumen-positive transepithelial voltage reduces the driving force for Mg^{2+} and Ca^{2+} reabsorption in the loop of Henle
Presentation
Approximately 50% of patients with ADH have associated hypomagnesemia
Bartter syndrome
Pathophysiology
Mutations in five ion transport proteins are described; all play a key role in transcellular Na^+ transport and generation of the lumen-positive voltage that is the driving force for Mg^{2+} and Ca^{2+} transport
Mutated transport genes include the Na^+-K^+-$2Cl^-$ cotransporter (NKCC2), the apical membrane K^+ channel (ROMK), the basolateral membrane Cl^- channel (ClC-Kb), barttin the β subunit of the basolateral membrane Cl^- channel, and severe gain of function mutations of the Ca^{2+}-Mg^{2+}-sensing receptor
Presentation
Presents with renal salt wasting, hypokalemic metabolic alkalosis, and increased renin and aldosterone concentrations

TABLE 11–9 (Continued)

The phenotype varies depending on the gene mutated

NKCC2 and ROMK mutations—associated with severe salt wasting, neonatal presentation, and nephrocalcinosis; for unclear reasons hypomagnesemia is not common

ClC-Kb mutations—present during adolescence and 50% have hypomagnesemia

Barttin mutations—associated with sensorineural deafness, hypomagnesemia has not been reported

Abbreviations: FHHNC, familial hypomagnesemia with hypercalciuria and nephrocalcinosis; ADH, autosomal dominant hypocalcemia; ROMK, renal outer medullary potassium

TABLE 11–10: Hypomagnesemia—Hereditary Renal Causes (Distal Convoluted Tubule, Figure 11–3)

IDH
Pathophysiology
IDH is due to a defect in the FXYD2 gene that encodes the γ subunit of the basolateral Na^+-K^+ ATPase in distal convoluted tubule
Mutations result in subunit retention in the Golgi complex
Presentation
An autosomal dominant disorder associated with hypocalciuria and chondrocalcinosis

Gitelman's syndrome
Pathophysiology
Results from loss of function mutations in the thiazide-sensitive NCCT
Mutant NCCT is trapped in the Golgi and not trafficked to the apical membrane
Presentation
Patients present in adolescence with symptoms of hypomagnesemia and almost always have associated hypocalciuria
Gitelman's syndrome results in more profound hypomagnesemia than is seen with chronic thiazide therapy

Abbreviations: IDH, isolated dominant hypomagnesemia; ATP, adenosine triphosphate; NCCT, NaCl cotransporter

TABLE 11–11: Hypomagnesemia—Caused by a Mitochondrial tRNA Mutation (Presumed DCT)

Pathophysiology

Affected fathers never transmit the trait, affected mothers transmit the trait to a high fraction of offspring consistent with mitochondrial inheritance

Result of a mutation in the mitochondrial tRNA^{Ile} gene

Presentation

Hypomagnesemia, hypertension, and hypercholesterolemia

Urinary FE of Mg^{2+} increased

Reduced urinary calcium excretion

Abbreviations: DCT, distal convoluted tubule; FE, fractional excretion

TABLE 11–12: Signs and Symptoms

It is difficult to attribute specific symptoms to hypomagnesemia due to its common association with metabolic alkalosis, hypocalcemia and hypokalemia

Increased neuromuscular excitability

Manifests as weakness, tetany, positive Chvostek's and Trousseau's signs, and seizures

A decreased concentration of either Mg^{2+} or Ca^{2+} can lower the threshold for nerve stimulation

Cardiovascular

Hypomagnesemia is associated with a variety of atrial and ventricular arrhythmias

Mg^{2+} affects several ion channels in heart; it regulates K^+ channels that open in the absence of Mg^{2+}

Mg^{2+} is a critical cofactor for the Na^+-K^+ ATPase and hypomagnesemia decreases pump activity; as a result, intracellular K^+ decreases with hypomagnesemia and depolarizes the cardiac myocyte resting membrane potential

The threshold for generation of an action potential is reduced and potential for arrhythmias increased

Decreased intracellular K^+ also decreases the speed of K^+ efflux resulting in a prolonged repolarization time

Hypomagnesemia aggravates digitalis toxicity since both decrease the activity of the Na^+-K^+ ATPase

Association with hypokalemia

Hypokalemia is frequently associated with hypomagnesemia

TABLE 11–12 (Continued)

Mg^{2+} is an inhibitor of apical membrane K^+ channels involved in K^+ secretion
A decrease in intracellular Mg^{2+} releases the inhibitory effect and increases K^+ secretion
Renal Mg^{2+} and K^+ losses may be unrelated but both occur in patients with specific diseases such as alcoholism, diabetic ketoacidosis, osmotic diuresis, and diuretic use
Association with hypocalcemia
Balance studies show that the hypocalcemia is not associated with a net negative Ca^{2+} balance indicating that it results from alterations in internal homeostatic mechanisms
Chronic hypomagnesemia suppresses PTH release from the parathyroid gland and this effect is rapidly reversed by intravenous Mg^{2+} infusion; this suggests that part of the effect is due to inhibition of PTH release
Hypomagnesemia-induced hypocalcemia may result from skeletal resistance to PTH; in vitro studies show that Mg^{2+} depletion interferes with PTH-stimulated cAMP generation
End-organ resistance occurs at serum Mg^{2+} concentrations ≤ 1.0 mg/dL
Serum Mg^{2+} concentrations ≤ 0.5 mg/dL are required to decrease PTH secretion

Abbreviations: ATP, adenosine triphosphate; PTH, parathyroid hormone; cAMP, cyclic adenosine monophosphate

TABLE 11–13: Approach to the Patient with Hypomagnesemia (Figure 11–4)
The two major sources of Mg^{2+} loss from the body are the GI tract and kidney
When Mg^{2+} losses are extrarenal the kidney will conserve Mg^{2+}
Evaluate renal magnesium handling
One can use the FE of Mg^{2+} (shown in Eq.11-1) or a 24-h urine to determine the kidney's response to hypomagnesemia
Renal Mg^{2+} excretion low-extrarenal etiology (GI cause or secondary to cell shifts)
The 24-h urinary Mg^{2+} excretion is less than 30 mg and FE of Mg^{2+} < 4%
• The most common GI causes are malabsorption and diarrhea; a careful history and physical examination should reveal these disorders
• Hypomagnesemia from decreased oral intake alone and primary intestinal hypomagnesemia are rare
• Mg^{2+} shifts from ECF to ICF are uncommon causes of hypomagnesemia but should be looked for after parathyroidectomy, refeeding, and in patients with hyperthyroidism
Renal Mg^{2+} excretion high-renal etiology
The 24-h urinary Mg^{2+} excretion is greater than 30 mg and the FE of Mg^{2+} greater than 4%

TABLE 11–13 (Continued)
Renal Mg^{2+} wasting is caused by primary defects in renal tubular reabsorption or secondary to systemic and local factors that the kidney is responding to
Drug- or toxin-induced injury is the most common cause of primary renal Mg^{2+} wasting
• A careful drug exposure history is obtained for aminoglycosides, *cis*-platinum, amphotericin B, pentamidine, cyclosporin, and cetuximab
• A variety of rare inherited renal Mg^{2+} wasting diseases should be considered (see Pathophysiology)
Systemic and local factors can affect Mg^{2+} reabsorption in proximal tubule, thick ascending limb of Henle, and distal tubule
• Osmotic diuresis reduces proximal tubule Mg^{2+} reabsorption
• Loop diuretics such as furosemide cause mild renal Mg^{2+} wasting due to an associated increase in proximal tubular Mg^{2+} reabsorption secondary to volume contraction
• Hypercalcemia results in renal Mg^{2+} wasting via effects on the Ca^{2+}-Mg^{2+}-sensing receptor
• Thiazide diuretics act in distal convoluted tubule to block Mg^{2+} transport; as with loop diuretics, their effect is mild due to enhanced proximal tubular Mg^{2+} reabsorption from ECF volume contraction
Normomagnesemic magnesium depletion
Serum Mg^{2+} concentration may not accurately reflect total body Mg^{2+} stores

(continued)

TABLE 11–13 (Continued)

In patients with unexplained hypocalcemia, hypokalemia, or symptoms of neuromuscular excitability the possibility of normomagnesemic Mg^{2+} depletion should be considered

In patients at high risk for Mg^{2+} depletion, a therapeutic trial of Mg^{2+} replacement may be warranted

Mg^{2+} replacement carries little risk provided renal function is normal

$$Fe_{Mg} = \frac{U_{Mg} \times P_{Cr}}{(0.7 \times P_{Mg}) \times U_{Cr}} \times 100 \qquad (11\text{-}1)$$

Abbreviations: GI, gastrointestinal; FE, fractional excretion; ECF, extracellular fluid; ICF, intracellular fluid

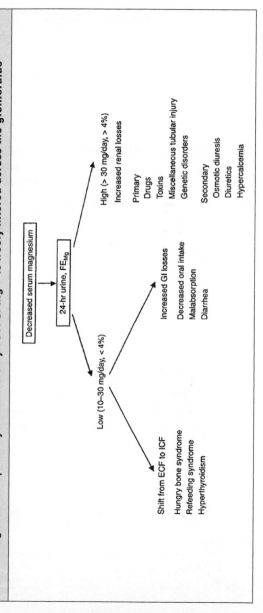

FIGURE 11–4: Approach to the Patient with Hypomagnesemia. If the diagnosis is not readily apparent from the history, either a 24-hour urine for Mg^{2+} or spot urine for calculation of the fractional excretion of Mg^{2+} is obtained. The fractional excretion of Mg^{2+} is calculated from equation 11.1. Serum Mg^{2+} is multiplied by 0.7 since only 70% of Mg^{2+} is freely filtered across the glomerulus

Decreased serum magnesium

24-hr urine, FE_{Mg}

High (> 30 mg/day, > 4%)
Increased renal losses

Primary
Drugs
Toxins
Miscellaneous tubular injury
Genetic disorders

Secondary
Osmotic diuresis
Diuretics
Hypercalcemia

Low (10–30 mg/day, < 4%)

Increased GI losses
Decreased oral intake
Malabsorption
Diarrhea

Shift from ECF to ICF
Hungry bone syndrome
Refeeding syndrome
Hyperthyroidism

TABLE 11–14: Treatment

General principles

The route of Mg^{2+} repletion varies depending on the severity of associated symptoms

Since renal Mg^{2+} excretion is regulated by the concentration sensed at the basolateral surface of the TALH, an acute infusion results in an abrupt increase in serum concentration and often a dramatic increase in renal Mg^{2+} excretion; for this reason much of intravenously administered Mg^{2+} is quickly excreted

Attempts are made to correct the underlying condition

Drugs that result in renal Mg^{2+} wasting should be minimized or discontinued

Life threatening symptoms—present

The acutely symptomatic patient with seizures, tetany, or ventricular arrhythmias related to hypomagnesemia should be administered Mg^{2+} intravenously

In the life-threatening setting 4 mL (2 ampules) of a 50% solution of magnesium sulfate diluted in 100 mL of normal saline (16 mEq of Mg^{2+}; 1 gm $MgSO_4$=8 m Eq Mg^{2+}) can be administered over 10 min; this is followed by 50 mEq of Mg^{2+} given over the next 12–24 h

The goal is to increase serum Mg^{2+} concentration above 1.0 mg/dL

Mg^{2+} is administered cautiously in patients with impaired renal function and serum concentration monitored frequently

TABLE 11–14 (Continued)
In the setting of chronic kidney disease the dose is reduced by 50–75%
Life threatening symptoms—absent
In the absence of a life-threatening condition Mg^{2+} is administered orally
Oral administration is more efficient because it results in less of an acute rise in serum Mg^{2+} concentration
Amiloride increases Mg^{2+} reabsorption in connecting tubule and collecting duct and may reduce renal Mg^{2+} wasting or decrease the dose of Mg^{2+} replacement if diarrhea becomes problematic
Amiloride is not used in patients with impaired renal function because of the risk of hyperkalemia
Abbreviations: TALH, thick ascending limb of Henle

TABLE 11–15: Treatment—Specific Cardiovascular Settings

Ventricular and atrial arrhythmias in the setting of an acute MI

Patients with mild hypomagnesemia in the setting of an acute MI have a two- to threefold increased incidence of ventricular arrhythmias in the first 24 h

This relationship persists for as long as 2–3 weeks after an MI

Mg^{2+} should be maintained in the normal range in this setting

Torsades de pointes and refractory ventricular fibrillation

The American Heart Association Guidelines for Cardiopulmonary Resuscitation recommend the use of IV Mg^{2+} for the treatment of torsades de pointes

Torsades de pointes (1–2 grams magnesium sulfate in 10 ml DSW over 5–20 min.) is a ventricular arrhythmia often precipitated by drugs that prolong the QT interval; Mg^{2+} does not shorten the QT interval and its effect may be mediated via Na^+ channel inhibition

After cardiopulmonary bypass

Hypomagnesemia is common after cardiopulmonary bypass and may result in an increased incidence of atrial and ventricular arrhythmias

Studies on prophylactic Mg^{2+} repletion in this setting are conflicting

Abbreviations: MI, myocardial infarction; IV, intravenous

TABLE 11–16: Oral Mg²⁺ Preparations

General principles

Slow release preparations of MgCl and Mg lactate are preferable since they cause less diarrhea

Diarrhea is the major side effect of Mg^{2+} repletion

25–100 mEq/day in divided doses is generally required

Preparation	MW	Formula	mg Mg^{2+}/gm	mEq Mg^{2+}/gm
Mg carbonate	84	$MgCO_3$	289	24
MgCl	203	$MgCl_2 \cdot 6H_2O$	119	10
Mg gluconate	415	$(CH_2OH(CHOH)_4COO)_2Mg$	58	5
Mg lactate	202	$Mg(C_3H_5O_3)_2$	120	10
Mg oxide	40	MgO	602	50
Mg sulfate	246	$MgSO_4 \cdot 7H_2O$	98	8

Abbreviation: MW, molecular weight

HYPERMAGNESEMIA

TABLE 11–17: Etiologies of Hypermagnesemia
The kidney can excrete virtually the entire filtered Mg^{2+} load in the presence of hypermagnesemia; for this reason hypermagnesemia is relatively uncommon unless high doses are administered intravenously or there is a decrease in glomerular filtration rate
IV Mg^{2+} load in the absence of CKD
Treatment of preterm labor
Treatment of eclampsia
Oral Mg^{2+} load in the presence of CKD
Laxatives
Antacids
Epsom salts
Miscellaneous
Salt water drowning
Abbreviations: IV, intravenous ; CKD, chronic kidney disease

TABLE 11–18: Hypermagnesemia—Pathophysiology and Presentation

It most often occurs with Mg^{2+} administration in the setting of a severe decrease in glomerular filtration rate

IV Mg^{2+} Load in the Absence of CKD

Pathophysiology

High doses of Mg^{2+} given intravenously can result in hypermagnesemia even in the absence of CKD

Presentation

The typical setting is obstetrical with Mg^{2+} infused for the management of preterm labor or eclampsia

Typical protocols often result in serum Mg^{2+} concentrations of 4–8 mg/dL

Oral Mg^{2+} Load in the Presence of CKD

The most common cause of hypermagnesemia is CKD

Pathophysiology

As glomerular filtration rate falls the fractional excretion of Mg^{2+} increases; this allows Mg^{2+} balance to be maintained until the glomerular filtration rate falls below 30 mL/min

Hypermagnesemia due to oral Mg^{2+} ingestion occurs most commonly in the setting of CKD

Presentation

Advanced age, CKD, and GI disturbances that enhance Mg^{2+} absorption such as decreased motility, gastritis, and colitis are contributing factors

- Cathartics, antacids, and Epsom salts are frequently the source of Mg^{2+}

(continued)

TABLE 11–18 (Continued)
Lithium intoxication and familial hypocalciuric hypercalcemia
• Presents with mild hypermagnesemia from decreased renal excretion
• This is due to the interaction of lithium with the basolateral Ca^{2+}-Mg^{2+}-sensing receptor in the TALH
• Antagonism of this receptor causes enhanced Mg^{2+} reabsorption
Miscellaneous
Salt water drowning
• Seawater is high in Mg^{2+} (14 mg/dL)
Abbreviations: IV, intravenous; CKD, chronic kidney disease; GI, gastrointestinal; TALH, thick ascending limb of Henle

TABLE 11–19: Signs and Symptoms

Signs and symptoms are primarily either neuromuscular or cardiac

Neuromuscular

Mg^{2+} blocks the synaptic transmission of nerve impulses; initially this results in lethargy and drowsiness

As Mg^{2+} concentration increases deep tendon reflexes are diminished (4–8 mg/dL)

Deep tendon reflexes are lost and mental status decreases at serum Mg^{2+} concentrations of 8–12 mg/dL

At Mg^{2+} concentrations >12 mg/dL flaccid paralysis and apnea occur

Parasympathetic blockage resulting in fixed and dilated pupils that mimics brainstem herniation was reported

Smooth muscle function can be affected resulting in ileus and urinary retention

Cardiac

Mg^{2+} blocks Ca^{2+} and K^+ channels required for action potential repolarization

At serum Mg^{2+} concentrations above 7 mg/dL hypotension and ECG changes such as PR prolongation, QRS widening, and QT prolongation are noted

At Mg^{2+} concentrations greater than 10 mg/dL ventricular fibrillation, complete heart block, and cardiac arrest occur

Abbreviation: ECG, electrocardiogram

TABLE 11–20: Diagnosis—Principles
Hypermagnesemia is often iatrogenic
A careful medication history is essential to determine the Mg^{2+} source, whether IV, as in the treatment of obstetrical disorders or oral
Laxatives, antacids, and Epsom salts are the most common oral Mg^{2+} sources; high doses of IV Mg^{2+} may result in hypermagnesemia in the absence of CKD
Hypermagnesemia from increased gastrointestinal Mg^{2+} absorption often requires some degree of renal impairment
The elderly are at increased risk, often because the degree of decrease in glomerular filtration rate is not adequately appreciated based on the serum creatinine concentration
The elderly often have decreased intestinal motility that further increases intestinal Mg^{2+} absorption
Abbreviations: IV, intravenous; CKD, chronic kidney disease; GI, gastrointestinal

TABLE 11–21: Treatment

Since the majority of cases of hypermagnesemia are iatrogenic, caution should be exercised in the use of Mg^{2+} salts especially in patients with CKD, those with GI disorders that may increase Mg^{2+} absorption, and the elderly

Excessive Mg^{2+} administration

The Mg^{2+} source should be identified and discontinued

Patients with CKD should be cautioned to avoid Mg^{2+}-containing antacids and laxatives

If the patient has hypotension or respiratory depression, Ca^{2+} (100–200 mg of elemental Ca^{2+} over 5–10 min) is administered intravenously

Increased renal Mg^{2+} excretion

Renal Mg^{2+} excretion is increased with a normal saline infusion and/or furosemide administration

In the patient with severe CKD or end-stage renal disease dialysis is often required

Hemodialysis is the modality of choice if the patient's hemodynamics can tolerate it, since it removes more Mg^{2+} than continuous venovenous hemofiltration or peritoneal dialysis

Abbreviations: CKD, chronic kidney disease; gastrointestinal; IV, intravenous

12
Appendix

INTRODUCTION

TABLE 12–1: Regulation of RPF and GFR
RPF and GFR are critical to a number of the kidney's homeostatic functions
Regulation of RPF and GFR occurs through changes in afferent and efferent arteriolar resistance
Autoregulation and TGF interact to maintain RPF and GFR constant
Abbreviations: RPF, renal plasma flow; GFR, glomerular filtration rate; TGF, tubuloglomerular feedback

TABLE 12–2: Autoregulation of Renal Blood Flow
Prevents large swings in RPF and GFR expected from changes in arterial perfusion pressure
Effects are mediated through changes in afferent arteriolar tone
• This maintains GFR constant until MAP < 70 mmHg or > 160 mmHg
• GFR ceases at a MAP < 40–50 mmHg
Myogenic stretch receptors in the afferent arteriolar wall play an important role in autoregulation
Autoregulation of the renal circulation maintains a relatively constant RPF and GFR
TGF mediates changes in GFR through alterations in solute delivery sensed by the macula densa
Abbreviations: RPF, renal plasma flow; GFR, glomerular filtration rate; MAP, mean arterial pressure; TGF, tubuloglomerular feedback

TABLE 12–3: TGF Mediates GFR Changes

Specialized macula densa cells, located at the end of the TALH, sense changes in tubular fluid Cl^- entry

Increases in renal perfusion increase GFR, which enhances NaCl delivery to the macula densa

Signaling at the macula densa results in vasoconstriction of the afferent arteriole and a reduction of GFR

This reduces glomerular capillary pressure (P_{GC}) and returns GFR toward normal and reduces NaCl delivery to the macula densa

Reduced NaCl delivery, as occurs with prerenal azotemia, has the opposite effect

Signaling at the macula densa results in vasodilation of the afferent arteriole and an increase in GFR

The mediator(s) of TGF are not well understood

- Adenosine and thromboxane

  - Increased when excessive Cl^- entry is sensed by macula densa (constricting afferent arteriole)

  - Reduced when Cl^- delivery is low, allowing afferent arteriolar vasodilatation

- Nitric oxide modulates TGF response to NaCl delivery; TGF is reset by variations in salt intake

  - Low NaCl delivery increases nitric oxide

  - Increased NaCl delivery reduces nitric oxide

Abbreviations: TGF, tubuloglomerular feedback; GFR, glomerular filtration rate; TALH, thick ascending limb of Henle

TABLE 12–4: Effect of Neurohormones on Autoregulation and TGF

Actions of systemic neurohormonal factors supersede autoregulation and TGF in certain disease states such as true or effective arterial blood volume depletion

Vasoconstrictor (SNS, RAAS, endothelin) and vasodilator (prostaglandins, nitric oxide) substances are produced

Renal vasoconstriction is balanced by the production of vasodilatory substances

- Prostaglandins (PGE_2, PGI_2) and nitric oxide

- NSAIDs tip balance in favor of vasoconstriction and reduce GFR in states where the SNS or the RAAS are activated

Abbreviations: TGF, tubuloglomerular feedback; SNS, sympathetic nervous system; RAAS, renin-angiotensin-aldosterone system; GFR, glomerular filtration rate; NSAIDs, nonsteroidal anti-inflammatory agents

CLINICAL ASSESSMENT OF GFR

TABLE 12–5: Normal GFR with Age	
GFR measurement is essential in patients with kidney disease	
Age adjusted normal GFR values are shown	
Age	**GFR (mL/min/1.73 m^2)**
5–7 days	51 ± 6
1–2 months	65 ± 6
5–8 months	88 ± 12
9–12 months	87 ± 8
≥18 months	124 ± 26 male, 109 ± 13 female
Abbreviation: GFR, glomerular filtration rate	

TABLE 12–6: Measures Available to Estimate Kidney Function
Serum creatinine concentration
Age adjusted normal GFR values (Table 12–5)
Creatinine clearance measurement (24-h urine)
Radiolabeled iothalamate
Creatinine clearance estimation (Cockcroft-Gault equation)
GFR estimation (MDRD equations)
Abbreviations: GFR, glomerular filtration rate; MDRD, Modification of diet in renal disease

TABLE 12–7: Serum Creatinine Concentration as a Measure of Kidney Function

Serum creatinine concentration is a common marker employed to estimate kidney function
It is produced from metabolism of skeletal muscle creatine
Creatinine enters urine via filtration and tubular secretion (organic cation transporter) in PCT
• Creatinine clearance overestimates GFR by 10–20%
• Creatinine secretion increases with declining GFR
Serum creatinine concentration alone is inaccurate and suboptimal to estimate GFR
In men and women, serum creatinine concentration rises little as GFR falls from 120 mL/min to 60 mL/min
Large changes in GFR result in minimal changes in serum creatinine concentration (increased tubular creatinine secretion)
Once GFR declines to 40–60 mL/min, tubular creatinine secretion is maximized
• Small changes in GFR result in large changes in serum creatinine concentration below this level
Abbreviations: PCT, proximal convoluted tubule; GFR, glomerular filtration rate

TABLE 12–8: Creatinine Clearance Measurement

Creatinine clearance is calculated by the formula shown below:

$$\text{CrCl (mL/min)} = [\text{UCr (mg/dL)} \times \text{Volume (mL/min)}] \div \text{PCr (mg/dL)} \qquad (12\text{-}1)$$

PCr is plasma creatinine concentration; UCr is 24-h urine creatinine concentration and volume is the total urine volume

Problems with 24-h urine include

- Creatinine clearance is an inaccurate measure of GFR (overestimates GFR)

- Cimetidine administration competitively blocks tubular cell creatinine secretion and enhances test accuracy

- Combining creatinine and urea clearance gives a close estimate at lower GFR levels

- Problems with patient collection of urine sample (under/overcollection)

Examining the ratio of creatinine to body weight in kilograms assesses the completeness of the collection

- Women should excrete 15–20 mg/kg of creatinine/day

- Men should excrete 20–25 mg/kg of creatinine/day

Abbreviation: GFR, glomerular filtration rate

TABLE 12–9: Formulas to Estimate Creatinine Clearance or GFR from Serum Creatinine Concentration

Radiolabeled iothalamate provides an accurate estimate of GFR; it is not widely available, and is expensive and cumbersome

Equations were created using serum creatinine concentration (and other data) to more accurately estimate creatinine clearance or GFR

- Cockcroft-Gault equation (estimates creatinine clearance)

$$([140 - age\ (years)] \times weight\ in\ kg$$
$$\div\ [72 \times serum\ creatinine\ (mg/dL)]$$
$$\times 0.85\ for\ females) \qquad (12\text{-}2)$$

- MDRD equations (accurately estimate GFR when < 60 mL/min)

  - *MDRD equation 7* requires BUN and serum albumin concentrations

$$(170 \times [serum\ creatinine\ (mg/dL)]^{-0.999}$$
$$\times [age\ (years)]^{-0.176} \times [0.762\ if\ female]$$
$$\times [1.18\ if\ African\text{-}American]$$
$$\times [BUN\ (mg/dL)]^{-0.170}$$
$$\times [albumin\ (g/dL)]^{+0.318}) \qquad (12\text{-}3)$$

  - *Abbreviated form of the MDRD equation* also accurately estimates GFR

$$(186 \times [serum\ creatinine\ (mg/dL)]^{-1.154}$$
$$\times [age\ (years)]^{-0.203} \times [0.742\ if\ female]$$
$$\times [1.21\ if\ African\text{-}American]) \qquad (12\text{-}4)$$

Abbreviations: GFR, glomerular filtration rate; BUN, blood urea nitrogen; MDRD, modification of diet in renal disease

TABLE 12–10: Ion Conversions

Sodium

1 gm = 43 mEq, 1 mEq = 23.25 mg, 1gm NaCl = 17 mEq Na$^+$

Potassium

1 mEq = 40.9 mg

Phosphorus

1 mmol/L = 3.12 mg/dL, 1 mmol = 31.25 mg

Calcium

Atomic weight—40.08, 1 mmol/L = 4 mg/dL, 1 mg/dL = 0.25 mmol/L

Magnesium

Atomic weight—24.3, 1 mmol = 24.3 mg, 1 mEq = 12 mg

Index

Note: Figures are indicated by *f* following the page reference